How to Look Expensive

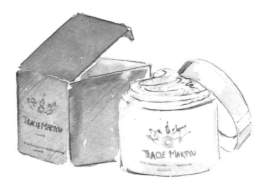

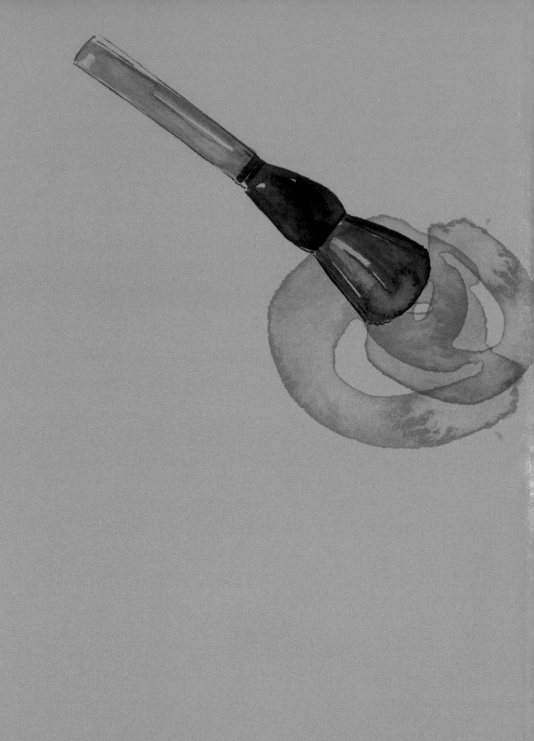

How to Look Expensive

A Beauty Editor's Secrets to Getting Gorgeous
without Breaking the Bank

ANDREA POMERANTZ LUSTIG

GOTHAM
BOOKS

GOTHAM BOOKS
Published by Penguin Group (USA) Inc.
375 Hudson Street, New York, New York 10014, U.S.A.
Penguin Group (Canada), 90 Eglinton Avenue East, Suite 700, Toronto, Ontario M4P 2Y3,
Canada (a division of Pearson Penguin Canada Inc.); Penguin Books Ltd, 80 Strand, London
WC2R 0RL, England; Penguin Ireland, 25 St Stephen's Green, Dublin 2, Ireland (a division of
Penguin Books Ltd); Penguin Group (Australia), 250 Camberwell Road, Camberwell, Victoria
3124, Australia (a division of Pearson Australia Group Pty Ltd); Penguin Books India Pvt Ltd,
11 Community Centre, Panchsheel Park, New Delhi–110 017, India; Penguin Group (NZ), 67
Apollo Drive, Rosedale, Auckland 0632, New Zealand (a division of Pearson New Zealand Ltd);
Penguin Books (South Africa) (Pty) Ltd, 24 Sturdee Avenue, Rosebank, Johannesburg 2196,
South Africa

Penguin Books Ltd, Registered Offices: 80 Strand, London WC2R 0RL, England

Published by Gotham Books, a member of Penguin Group (USA) Inc.

First printing, August 2012
10 9 8 7 6 5 4 3 2 1

An extension of this copyright page can be found on pages 208–209.

Illustrations on the following pages by Aimee Levy/Art Department: 15, 17, 19, 21, 23, 34, 35,
40, 41, 59, 114, 121, 122, 124, 126, 134, 135, 139, 164, 185

Illustrations on the following pages by Dallas Shaw: i, ii, v, vi, viii, xii, 8, 12, 25, 28, 31, 32, 33, 45,
46, 48, 55, 56, 65, 66, 70, 73, 76, 78, 79, 81, 87, 93, 99, 100, 102, 107, 108, 109, 112, 117, 119, 125,
127, 129, 133, 140, 142, 143, 149, 150, 163, 166, 167, 177, 179, 180, 187, 189, 190, 192, 194, 196,
199, 202

Gotham Books and the skyscraper logo are trademarks of Penguin Group (USA) Inc.

LIBRARY OF CONGRESS CATALOGING-IN-PUBLICATION DATA
Lustig, Andrea Pomerantz.
How to look expensive : a beauty editor's secrets to getting gorgeous without breaking the bank
/ Andrea Pomerantz Lustig.
p. cm.
ISBN 978-1-592-40723-1 (pbk.)
1. Beauty, Personal. 2. Cosmetics. 3. Skin Care and hygiene I. Title.
RA778.L953   2012
646.7'2—dc23   2011051639

Printed in the United States of America
Set in Utopia STD
Designed by Hoffman Creative

While the author has made every effort to provide accurate telephone numbers and Internet
addresses at the time of publication, neither the publisher nor the author assumes any
responsibility for errors, or for changes that occur after publication. Further, the publisher does
not have any control over and does not assume any responsibility for author or third-party
websites or their content.

TO ANNA

Now that you and your friends have discovered my stash
of products, I hope you'll take my advice on how to use them.
Not that you need them. I love you.

TO MATTHEW, MICHAEL, AND JAMES

I don't mention it inside this book, but there's no greater
beauty secret than surrounding yourself with love.
It's priceless. And I love you for it.

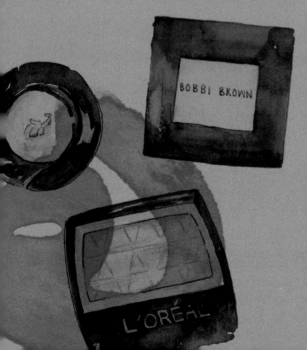

Contents

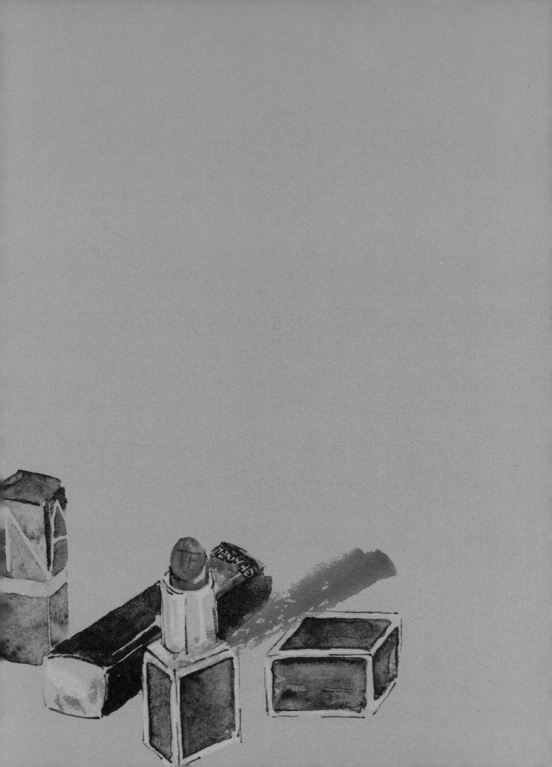

You are holding in your hands a book filled with the kind of insider beauty information celebrities pay top dollar to get. It's by one of the top writers in the business. Every page delivers. There's only one problem.

I wish she had written it ten years ago!

Ever since I met Andrea, I have been hoping that she would sit down, take out her laptop, and write down some—not even all, just some!—of the encyclopedic beauty knowledge that lines her brain. Her *Glamour* columns, features, and blog posts on everything from face masks to growing out layers are deliciously satisfying, but as someone who's had the privilege of editing her for a decade, I knew there was *so much more*. Ask her any question about your looks and Andrea will have the perfect, no-BS, highly informed answer, which, if you're smart and you listen, will make you look a whole lot better by tomorrow morning. (If the answer involves a particular hair pro or makeup guy, she will also take out her iPhone, call that expert on Beyoncé's yacht, and get you an appointment.) Plus, she just *knows stuff*. When I picture the inside of Andrea Pomerantz Lustig's head, it looks like a cross between the Bergdorf Goodman beauty department and Mr. Magorium's Wonder Emporium, lined with little magic bottles, big books of potions, and that thing that is going to finally make my cowlick settle down after all these years.

So now she's done it. At last. And even if I kind of wish I'd had all these answers sooner, I forgive her. After all, she has the best possible motive: to help us all look "expensive," as she puts it, on *any* paycheck.

Before you dive in, it might help you to know a little about who Andrea is. If the word *expensive* makes you picture an overly made-up lady swanning about in a fur coat, let's grind to a screeching halt here. As Andrea will tell you, that's not the look she's talking about. And it's not *her*, either.

> *When I picture the inside of Andrea Pomerantz Lustig's head, it looks like a cross between the Bergdorf Goodman beauty department and Mr. Magorium's Wonder Emporium.*

Not that she's not glamorous. Andrea was literally the first person I met, ever, at *Glamour*; she interviewed me for an editorial assistant job she was vacating because she'd been promoted to Fancy Beauty Something. I was from Virginia and had never seen highlights, and Andrea's—even back then, in the Paleolithic era, before everyone had highlights—were top-of-the-line, glinting under the fluorescent lights of the conference room. She also had—was that a manicure? No one I knew got manicures, unless they were getting married the next day. Andrea hired me and promptly became my role model, not just in how to write and edit, but also in how to look like I had it together beautywise. She was the first person to get me hooked on foundation brushes (see page 108) and is the reason I currently spritz fragrance on my hairbrush rather than directly on my skin (see page 194); your boyfriend/husband, like mine, will find this hilarious, but it delivers exactly the right amount of scent.

But she was also, I quickly realized, a natural reporter. Andrea has a journalist's eye in a beauty editor's body: She knows what's new, understands what works, and can sniff out hype a mile away—and over the years, as Andrea became a columnist for *Glamour*, I understood how valuable her curiosity was. Andrea will see a celebrity looking ever so slightly different and hunt down the exact new product used to give that glow. She'll share what she loves but also blow the whistle on products and procedures that aren't worth your money (including, as she'll tell you here, over-Botoxing—"there's lots of potential to look weird," she writes).

> *Andrea has a journalist's eye in a beauty editor's body: She knows what's new, understands what works, and can sniff out hype a mile away.*

And she is a busy workwoman herself, running the same daily marathon as the rest of us, albeit generally in four-inch Louboutins and without visibly sweating. The heart and soul of her life are her husband and three kids, and she doesn't believe in anything that requires days at the salon to achieve or a small fortune to procure. She uses Starbucks napkins as face blotters (something about their texture is perfect, she swears) and claims not to even own perfume (she prefers fragranced lotions for a subtler effect). If you peek into her makeup drawer at home—Andrea, you had me over; what did you think I was going to do?—you'll find super-pricey skin creams next to drugstore finds that cost in the single digits.

And *that* is the reason millions of women have followed Andrea's columns and features over the years. Readers love her inside knowledge of the beauty biz; without her, I would never have known that celebs spray tan before long flights so the color settles in midflight and they can emerge before the airport paparazzi looking sun kissed, not sleep deprived like you and me. But it's the *shortcuts* to that luxe, high-end celebrity look that keep Andrea's fans hooked—and that's what this book is all about.

Andrea's version of expensive requires neither a Beverly Hills dermatologist nor membership in America's 1 percent, but you may look as if you have both before she's done with you.

I'm in. I bet you will be, too.

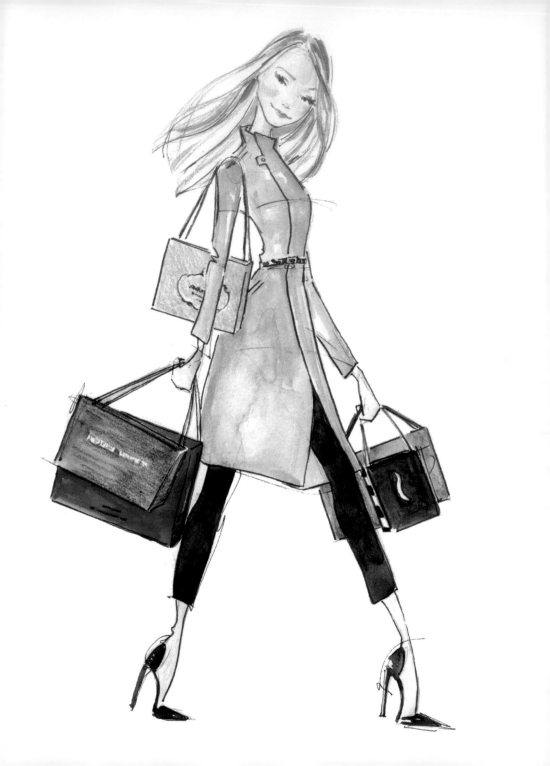

How to Look Expensive

————————— *An Introduction* —————————

Having spent most of my adult life giving women beauty advice, I know that how you look affects how you feel. And though it's not rocket science or nanotechnology, beauty matters. When you upgrade your look, you are setting yourself up to upgrade your life. To help you understand where I'm going, consider this: When a celebrity gets her first big role, she enters the Hollywood roller coaster of red-carpet events and 24-7 paparazzi coverage. It takes her a lot of time (and a lot of cash) to look as star-like off-screen as she does on-screen. But once the hair and makeup big guns get ahold of her, she begins to upgrade her look. And the more successful she gets, the more she spends looking the part. That's what I want to do for you . . . minus the price tag. I want to help you upgrade your image, stage your own "celebrity makeover." This book gives you access to hundreds of thousands of dollars of beauty advice that I hope will change your life, or at least make you look and feel like a million bucks.

When I tell people I've written a beauty advice column for *Glamour* for ten years (on top of having been the beauty editor of *Cosmopolitan* for the ten years before that!), first they get jealous, then they start bombarding me with questions about *all* of their beauty problems. I get asked about everything: puffy eyes, pimples, fading lipstick, runny eye makeup, Restylane, wrinkles, moisturizers, hair products, hair color, Latisse, lash extensions . . . you name it. They think I'm a walking encyclopedia of beauty knowledge and, truthfully, I guess I am. That's because I've spent my career living, breathing, touching, and studying just about every beauty product on the planet. And that's not even the most fun part of my job!

As a beauty journalist and the original *Glamour* beauty blogger, I've developed an awesome Rolodex of A-list hair and makeup artists who ring me up with their celebrity beauty scoop almost as soon as it happens. I have close relationships with these artists—visiting them at their studios, breaking for coffee with them backstage at fashion shows, and trading tips with them over Skype, Facebook chat, or cell phone. By now I'm sure you get the picture that I'm sitting on a GOLD MINE of beauty advice; this book is filled with the priceless beauty stories and tips I've gleaned along the way.

Of course actresses get all this pricey primping paid for by their movie companies, or else they can write off beauty services as a business expense (looking like a million bucks every time they walk out the door is, after all, a job for them). But how much would it cost a *real* woman to get the mega-exclusive, super–high-end beauty advice I get every day from my stylist pals? We're talking $$$$$$$$$$$$$$ GAZILLIONS, girls!

These days we're all much more money-conscious than we were before. Spending a bundle on your hair doesn't seem so sensible when filling your tank with gas costs more than a haircut. And this means there is a huge disconnect between the price of beauty and the money real women can actually spend on it. Not to mention the hyper–high-end beauty ideal we've grown

By now I'm sure you get the picture that I'm sitting on a GOLD MINE of beauty advice; this book is filled with the priceless beauty stories and tips I've gleaned along the way.

It's luxe, not loud. More Paris, France, than Paris Hilton.

accustomed to as gorgeous A-list actresses glam up just to go to the supermarket (with paparazzi trailing 24-7, I don't blame them!), and grace every magazine cover looking better and better even as they age (hello, Julianne Moore!). Even our first lady has her own hair and makeup team, the first presidential wife to do so. Surely this must be setting a new standard for the rest of us! And this led me to my EUREKA! moment: I can help bridge the gap between how we *want* to look and how we can *afford* to look by sharing my "wealth" of beauty knowledge—the tips, tricks, and techniques culled from both my beauty BFFs and the twenty-plus years I've spent collecting, testing, seeing, and hearing the world's best beauty advice.

Now I want to stop here and share a bit of my personal beauty philosophy to assure you that this book is not all about being vain and looking super wealthy (how shallow!) despite the title. I've always believed that improving your looks is a way to improve your life. Looking the part is part of getting the job, getting the promotion, getting the guy, having your best life. Sure, you can say I specialize in information that plenty of unknowing people might find irrelevant—lipstick, blush, pimples—but feeling like a million bucks makes you look like a million bucks. I swear it's true, and it's what keeps me at it. Why? Because I believe that beauty is power. When your hair looks polished, you feel polished. When you get your skin under control, you feel more in control of your life. The right lipstick color can lift your mood better than Prozac.

I also think it's important to take a closer look at my title, *How to Look Expensive*. Notice that I didn't call it *How to Look Loaded* or even *How to Look Rich*. That was very deliberate because to me, looking expensive is about looking chic and understated, polished and professional, your personal best. It's not about being flashy or a show-off or showgirl (that's a different kind of expensive). It's luxe, not loud. More Paris, France, than Paris Hilton.

The New Expensive:
Four Ways to Look Luxe

I truly believe there are many ways to look expensive, and throughout this book I'll give you examples of how to tailor my advice for your specific style. Take a look at these examples to see which look fits your personality best. Or keep a few in mind because it's okay to switch off between my different luxe personas just like some celebrities do, maybe favoring one type at work, another when you go out at night, and another for your own personal red-carpet events, or even rotating them based on your mood or environment. I for one can find myself in all of these looks!

PARK AVENUE PRETTY

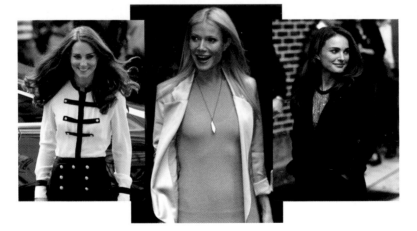

This is the classic, always-appropriate expensive look that embodies the spirit of a chic girl from New York's Upper East Side. Perfectly coiffed, shiny hair that looks like it was just blow-dried, which may or may not be true. Flawless makeup you know must be there, but you can hardly see it. In the last decade this look has undergone its own makeover, staying classic but becoming more current. Gone are the pearls and black silk headbands, and in their place is a statement

Think: *Kate Middleton, Gwyneth Paltrow, Natalie Portman, Kate Winslet, Anne Hathaway, Jennifer Aniston, Julianne Moore, Chanel Iman, Olivia Palermo*

necklace or bold nail color, no chips, of course. Movie stars who take an understated approach to glam fall into this category. They're the girls who wear a chic but understated gown on the red carpet instead of the of-the-moment, metallic, one-shouldered look-at-me number.

HOLLYWOOD BOHO

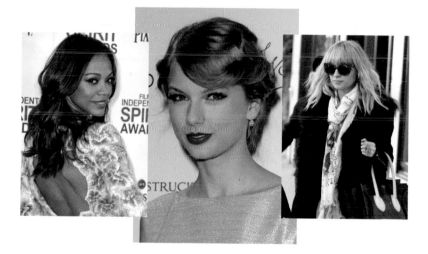

Think: *Zoe Saldana, Taylor Swift, Nicole Richie, Alexa Chung, Chloë Sevigny, Jessica Alba, Kate Hudson, Drew Barrymore, Elizabeth Olsen, Rihanna, Kristen Stewart, Christina Hendricks*

This downtown hipster oozes luxe in a very cool, effortless way. She's not unkempt or overly trendy but a total individual who makes her own bold statement. Her style is more boho than bad girl, kind of like the makeover Nicole Richie's gone through herself. She makes messy hair look chic, not like she forgot to brush it. She tends to play up her features very originally as her statement, be it a wash of totally not-gaudy silver eye shadow, elongated black eyeliner, an asymmetrical layered haircut, or an offbeat lip color, but still shows restraint and stays "pretty." That's what keeps the look from veering off to funky or punky instead of luxe. Picture Taylor Swift on the red carpet: Her movie-star bold mouth is always fuchsia, not red; her cat-eyeliner navy, not black; and her curly updos are just off-balance enough to look cool, not prim and proper or stuck-up.

GLAM GLOBE-TROTTER

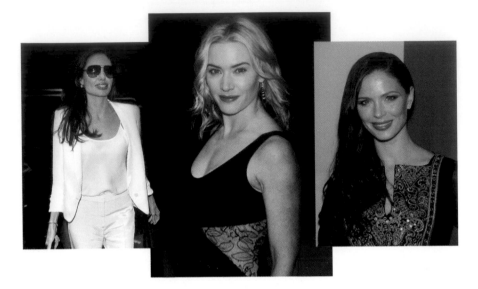

She's the world-traveling goddess who looks so effortlessly chic, you'd think she woke up gorgeous. She's queen of the neutral, no-color makeup look, but she never looks pale or washed out. Her hair doesn't require much effort and never looks over-styled. She's classic in a modern, Euro-chic kind of way—the kind of woman who can walk off an overnight flight looking no worse for the wear (and with still-perfect hair!).

Think: *Angelina Jolie, Kate Winslet, Georgina Chapman, Gisele Bündchen, Keira Knightley, Mila Kunis, Miranda Kerr, Kate Moss, Marion Cotillard, Sienna Miller*

THE RICH BITCH

There's one category of luxe look I won't recommend, and that's the trying-too-hard-to-look-like-a-rich-girl look! These are girls who try to look rich, but end up looking cheap. (Paris Hilton, Lindsay Lohan, Tara Reid, and Christina Aguilera come to mind.) Remember, looking high-end is all about subtlety, not showing off how much money you have! Lots of women make this mistake when they go to the hair colorist, demanding to see the color they paid for when, actually, good hair color looks natural. Is this starting to make sense?

MODERN MOVIE STAR

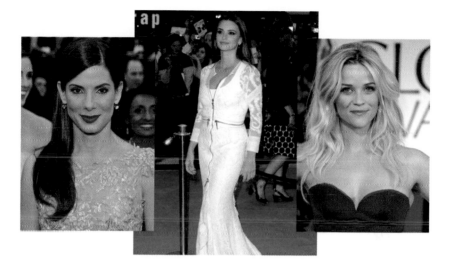

Think: *Sandra Bullock, Penelope Cruz, Reese Witherspoon, Scarlett Johansson, Jennifer Lopez, Sofia Vergara, January Jones, Eva Longoria*

This is the rags-to-riches kind of expensive, the girl who looks totally normal by day, you may not even recognize her if you saw her on the street, but who knows how to turn it on, big-time, by night. The red lipstick. The Veronica Lake waves. The shimmer that catches the light. The vavavoom white, champagne, lilac, peacock blue, or red-hot gown! Sure, she's a more contrived kind of expensive, but she never overdoes it, classic in a stylish way, just the girl you want to be when you have your own special event.

One more thing…

Before we move on I want to point out that having the high cheekbones or hefty checkbook of a celebrity isn't necessary to get the look I'm talking about. My goal is to help you look your best so you can be your best. And that's what the tips in the next chapters will help you do.

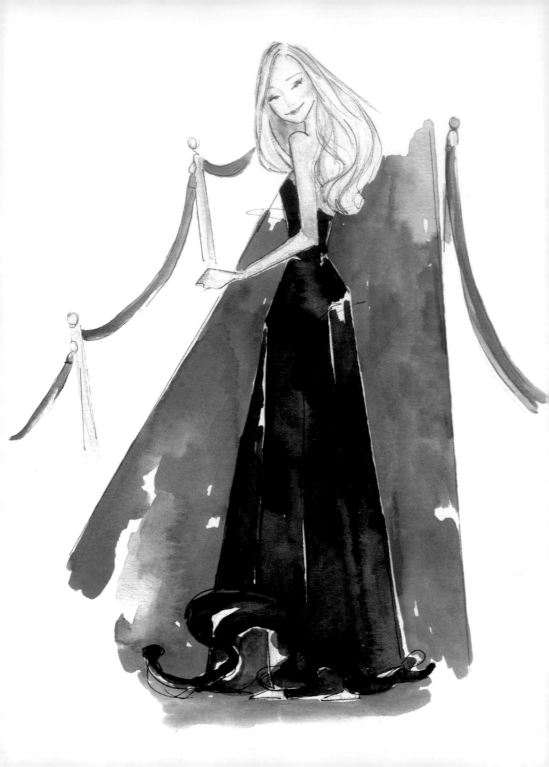

1

Your Hair

———— *A Wearable Status Symbol* ————

Expensive hair. You know it when you see it on someone else: the model with lustrous hair on a TV commercial or in a magazine spread who makes you want to reach out and touch the screen or the page; the actress on the red carpet with hair that sparkles almost as brightly as the million dollars' worth of diamonds hanging on her neck; Kate Middleton just being Kate Middleton, her royal mane flowing as she walks, giving me hope for the future Windsor family gene pool! Expensive hair is touchable, it moves, it reflects light, it looks alive, healthy.

Cheap hair on the other hand? It's hair that isn't healthy, doesn't move, isn't touchable, and doesn't catch the light. It's too teased, too layered, too poufed—what used to be called mall hair but now might be called Jersey Shore hair! It's split ends. Crunchy texture. Greasy roots. And funnily enough, it's also snotty socialite hair that looks too styled, like you're trying too hard (more on that later).

I don't think any woman sets out to look this way, but it often happens inadvertently. Women unknowingly overdo their hair with too much of everything—too much product, too much teasing, too much layering, too much heat. And cheap hair can happen no matter how fat your wallet. In fact, women with plenty of money are often the worst offenders. Truly, taste doesn't always come with a Platinum Card. Remember the Rich Bitch look we talked about earlier?

The Truth Behind the Great Hair You See in the Press

So why does every star in Hollywood have gorgeous, expensive-looking hair? They don't. It just looks that way. There's a fortune being spent on the hair you see and admire in the public eye—not to mention a lot of hair extensions! No wonder you can't compete. These stars are upping the ante for the rest of us, from the thousands that studios spend on top actresses' tresses for premieres and events to the big money that hair care companies invest at New York Fashion Week to the glamorization of hair on TV. Blake Lively is the perfect example of where this last trend can lead. Her gorgeous mane on *Gossip Girl* captured the attention of *Vogue* editors and Karl Lagerfeld, eventually scoring Blake the crème de la crème of endorsements, a Chanel contract! Even though the brand doesn't offer hair products, there's no denying Blake's bouncy, beautiful, expensive-looking flaxen mane helps sell plenty of Chanel handbags and cosmetics. But let's get back to where all this insider hair information leaves you, besides wondering if maybe you should quit your job and become a high-paid hairstylist.

Like most women, you're probably inwardly craving expensive hair yourself, wanting it, *dye*-ing for it, buying every shampoo on the planet to make it happen. The good news is you really *can* learn to be your own celebrity hairstylist. May I offer up my own transformation? I can't tell you

Cheap hair can happen no matter how fat your wallet.

how bad I was at DIYing my hair when I first became a beauty editor, but over the years, and through my relationships with the celebrity hair gurus, I've collected the secrets that make hair look gorgeously luxe. Many of them are small, important tweaks and details to add to what you already know how to do; some of the techniques are challenging until you practice them again and again. A hairstylist can do ten to twenty or more heads a day—that's a lot of practice. So read on, go for it, and practice, practice, practice. What's the worst that can happen? You hate your hair and put it in a ponytail? The next day, get right back behind the blow-dryer and try again. It might not take you to Carnegie Hall or the Cannes Film Festival, but once you experience that euphoric feeling you get when you love your hair (what I like to call "hair happiness"), you'll be hooked.

I've collected the secrets that make hair look gorgeously luxe.

HOW TO GET AN INEXPENSIVE (EVEN FREE!) HAIRCUT AT AN EXPENSIVE SALON!

- **Do "marketing" for your salon.** Ask your stylist for business cards and make a deal for a free haircut for every two new clients you bring in.

- **Like your salon** (or any salon you wish you could afford) on Facebook. And then pay attention for posts on specials and discounts. Also check out StyleSeat.com, Lifebooker, Gilt.com, Groupon, and other appointment-booking and online sale sites for specials.

- **Cry poor.** Seriously. Some stylists will work with you by either adjusting the price until you're back on your feet, or adjusting the haircut so you won't need maintenance as frequently.

- **Keep your hair longer.** The cut will last longer. Mine is past my shoulders and I can get away with two cuts a year.

- **Be a hair model.** Chichi salons usually have educational nights or classes for assistants and junior stylists. You can sign up for a free haircut supervised by a top stylist. Be sure to ask if you'll have a choice on the cut, length, or style (sometimes you won't).

How to Get a $500 Haircut at a $50 Salon

So you don't live in New York or LA and, even if you do, you can't afford a pricey salon bill. What's a girl to do? Her research! Just like Kate Middleton uncovers luxe-looking fashion at low-end London chain stores, you can find an affordable stylist who gives high-end haircuts.

- **Post a query on your Facebook page** or troll the stylists on StyleSeat.com, a website where stylists post their philosophies, galleries of looks they've created and online specials. It also lets you read testimonials, book appointments, and take advantage of special prices and promotions.

- **Read online reviews** on sites like Yelp.com and Lifebooker.com.

- **Ask friends** whose hair you admire where they go.

- **Stop a woman on the street** if you love her hair.

- **Visit an affordable salon**—in person or virtually on their website or on StyleSeat.com, and check out the stylists' work and see which one creates looks closest to what you want. Look at the stylist's own hair, makeup, and the way he or she dresses to see if your styles mesh.

Expensive hair enhances who you are, it doesn't define you.

Before your stylist begins, share your "absolute" list.

Once you've found a stylist, prepare for your visit with photos and images of hair you love (and hair you hate). Clip a photo from a magazine or google a celeb whose hair you crave and print out a picture. But before your stylist begins, share your "absolute" list. What you absolutely *must* have or absolutely *must not* have. For instance, stylist Creighton Bowman tells me he has a list of absolutes for each of his celeb clients. He knows if they must have a sideswept bang or a super-side part, if they hate it when their bangs are too long or so short they show their eyebrows—then whatever style he creates, he can work the absolutes in or out. Here's my absolute list: Body on the sides, not on top, an in-between part, left of center. Ends that flip back out instead of in and under. What's your absolute list? You've got to know it to find hair happiness from even the most expensive stylist.

The New Definition of Expensive When It Comes to Modern Hair

"In different eras, socialite hair was your moment at the salon, a time for women to socialize and get together during the weekly blow-dry or roller set, the goal being 'to look like I spent money on my hair.' Today, I think what looks expensive is a good haircut," says David Babaii, stylist to the stars and a good friend. (More from David coming up.) It's the difference between a wealthy reality-television wife and an A-list movie star. For the latter, gorgeous hair is just one subtle aspect of her look, while on the former, you notice almost nothing but her hair. It's just as showy as the giant diamond on her finger.

Remember: Expensive hair enhances who you are, it doesn't define you.

Five High-End Haircuts to Take to Your $50 Stylist

I want to introduce you to some friends of mine, the pros who spend their time coiffing the most prestigious manes in Hollywood. Imagine you're Anne Hathaway or Natalie Portman (or insert your favorite actress) and get ready for some priceless advice on what works best for your hair. You can take any one of these five fabulous, modern cuts to your own moderately priced salon and ask them to replicate the look!

BOOK AN APPOINTMENT WITH...

DAVID BABAII
The Hollywood Hair Star

Lucky David Babaii's first client was Kate Hudson. Actually his second client. Fresh out of beauty school, he met her PR person through a friend and gave him a haircut. Kate's publicist called the next day and booked David for a photo shoot with Kate. As David tells it: "Kate and I fell in love. I did her hair for the Oscars two days later and then my career went immediately through the roof, with Gwyneth and Angelina as clients three and four." Today his roster of celebrities would leave you starstruck.

"For most women, hair is a form of seduction, the ultimate accessory. They use it as protection."
—David Babaii

Babaii's Cheap Trick

The fake bob. Here's the technique that when worn by Scarlett Johansson, Uma Thurman, and Nicole Kidman sent paparazzi and beauty editors into a tizzy looking for the haircut scoop.

"Roll your long hair under and secure with bobby pins," says David. "For more drama, change the part first. Everyone will think you cut your hair!"

THE NO-HAIRCUT HAIRCUT

by David Babaii

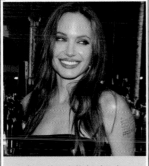

Angelina Jolie's simple yet sophisticated circle cut

This round-layered cut, the simple but sophisticated seventies-inspired haircut he gives Angelina Jolie, Nicole Kidman, and Kate Hudson, is one length all the way around. It's an all-time favorite of Babaii's because it's versatile and will last forever. "It's the perfect haircut if you can't afford to get your hair cut every six weeks," he says. Proof that less is always more, this is a classic, low-key cut that'll give long hair a modern, elegant look, just by tweaking the ends.

1. CIRCLE CUT

While establishing the length you want (any length will work with this cut), ask your stylist if he or she is familiar with the famous **Vidal Sassoon Circle Cut** to help visualize this look.

2. CURVE

Have your stylist pull a section of hair straight up from the roots, starting from the center at the top of the head. The center length will be your guidepost. He then should cut the edges of the section on a slight curve.

Keep going around the head, pulling up and cutting a new section to continue the curve. If you turn upside down, you should see a halo of hair surrounding your head like a perfect sphere. This creates almost invisible layers and an arched effect that will give ends rich-looking body and movement when dry.

TO STYLE

Try any style in this book or any style you want with this hair. Up, down, straight, curled, waved, this is the most versatile haircut. Period.

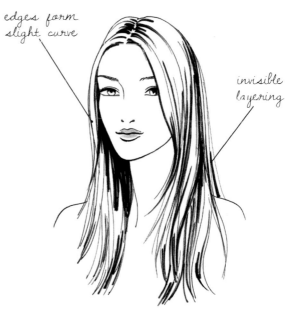

edges form slight curve

invisible layering

BOOK AN APPOINTMENT WITH...

ADIR ABERGEL
The Oscar Hairdresser

Once you've secured that Oscar nomination, call your mother. The next call to make? Your hairdresser. And if you think you might actually win, you better dial up Adir Abergel. A former dancer who left ballet school to become a stylist, he's now one of the most in-demand stylists in Hollywood, with a Frédéric Fekkai spokesperson contract to boot. Abergel, classic beauty Anne Hathaway's mane man, is all about touchable, feminine, rich-looking hair that's chic to the max, but not over styled.

"Less product, less product, less product. Hair looks more expensive when there's less gook in it."
—Adir Abergel

Adir's Cheap Tricks

A toothbrush sprayed with hair spray can be used to smooth out the front hairline and strands sticking up on the top of the head.

Be miserly with hair products. Adir suggests using product at the finish instead of the start, and says most women don't know this secret to using any hair product successfully: Spread it on your hands like a hand cream, emulsify it by rubbing your hands together, and then start underneath the hair, near the scalp, and run your fingers through your hair. This will help get the product evenly distributed instead of deposited right on top of your head where it can look greasy.

THE SEXY SHOULDER-SKIMMING CUT

by Adir Abergel

Adir's signature cut is the long-layered shoulder-length cut with side-sweeping long bangs that he gives all his girls (e.g., Sienna Miller, Anne Hathaway, Jennifer Garner). The shorter pieces add some movement around the face and the light layering gives the sides and bottom movement, too. It's the perfect mid-length cut that's anything but middle of the road—a super-luxe, super-sexy choice that's easy to manage and always looks expensive.

1. CENTER-PART HAIR

before you cut it so you can later part it on either side and get a great effect.

2. CUT THE OVERALL LENGTH FIRST.

In the front, create an angle by starting right above the jawline and angling the entire length of the front pieces. This will keep the front about one inch shorter than the back.

3. ADD LAYERS,

mostly around the face. In the back, keep the layering very slight (no more than two inches above the ends).

TO STYLE

Since this is a very diverse cut, you can either blow-dry it or wear it wash-and-go without using any heating devices.

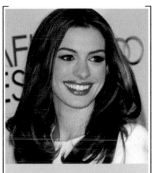

Adir's signature cut on Anne Hathaway

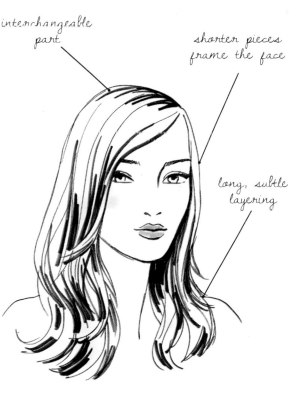

interchangeable part

shorter pieces frame the face

long, subtle layering

BOOK AN APPOINTMENT WITH...

CREIGHTON BOWMAN
The New York Hair Hipster

Creighton is based in New York but he's barely there. Instead he's usually jet-setting around the globe with his celebrity clientele. His hair is often inspired by Italian and French movie stars of the sixties and seventies (like Sophia Loren and Brigitte Bardot) and tends to be what he calls glamorous, sophisticated, and, at the same time, natural. Think Julia Roberts and Megan Fox. Both are Creighton's regulars.

"There's nothing classier than a bob, and this chic take incorporates subtle layering just on the ends, hitting the collarbone with a face-framing fringe."

—Creighton Bowman

Creighton's Cheap Tricks

Use corn starch baby powder as dry shampoo. "It's the base of many dry shampoos anyway, and it comes in an easy-to-use sprinkle container. I pour a little in my hands, clap them together, then rub my hands together and then through the hair."

Make your own texturizing spray. Creighton concocts his own salt spray for a beachy wave look by adding a few teaspoons of sea salt to a bottle of leave-in conditioner. Spritz over damp hair for a beachy wave look.

THE POSH AND PRETTY BOB

by Creighton Bowman

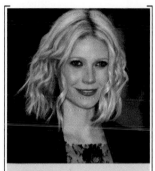

Gwyneth Paltrow's bob can go sleek or wavy.

This is a classic cut similar to the long bob Gwyneth made famous. You'll never get bored with it, and it's not too short for a ponytail.

1. ASK YOUR STYLIST for an A-line bob that is shorter in back, longer in front. The best length is no shorter than your natural hairline in back and no shorter than your jawbone in the front.

2. CUT LONG BANGS on an angle from the bridge of your nose to the top of your cheekbones. This will keep your cut from looking too boxy.

3. ADD LONG LAYERS to the tips to "bevel" the ends for softness. This will prevent the bob from getting too square and looking harsh.

TO STYLE
Blow-dry it straight for a sleek, modern look. Finish with a shine spray or oil for super sheen. At home, you've got lots of options: Dry it straight, air-dry with a beach or texturizing spray for soft waves, or add sexy curls at night.

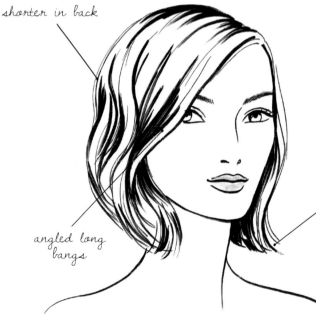

shorter in back

angled long bangs

beveled ends

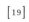

BOOK AN APPOINTMENT WITH...

HARRY JOSH
The Downtown Darling

Adorable Harry is famous for hair that looks casually chic and sexy in the way of an off-duty model (he calls his specialty MOD hair, Model Off Duty). He's the man to give you the kind of cool-girl locks you might see on the stylish streets of Manhattan's Meatpacking District, where he perches himself between worldwide assignments at the Serge Normant at John Frieda salon. If you're looking for understated chic hair with a cool factor, Harry's your man. The one look Harry won't do: the uptown hyper-polished, perfectly coiffed blow-out.

"I don't do the coiffed hair thing. It's just not who I am as a hairdresser. I think hair with a salon stamp all over it actually comes off as insecure, like you're trying to prove something."

—Harry Josh

DIY HARRY JOSH'S MOD HAIR

Best for straight hair or hair with a moderate natural wave/curl.

1. Wash your hair the night before. Sleep with it in a bun.

2. Wake up, take out the bun. Wrap hair in a towel while you shower.

3. Use dry shampoo to thicken hair if needed. Put some in your hands and rub it through the underneath layers of hair.

4. Brush hair from underneath so you don't take the wave out.

5. Use a curling iron to add more wave if you want it.

6. Leave hair down or tie back up into an undone bun. Let pieces fall out naturally in front for some face-framing prettiness.

Harry's Cheap Trick
Use a spritz bottle filled with water to mist over a style to make it look more lived-in or to reactivate product that's already in the hair instead of adding more.

Harry's Pet Peeve
Women in his chair who yack away on the cell phone or want to gossip instead of paying attention and then get home, call him, and say, "I have no idea how to do my hair." Instead, think of your hair appointment as a session with a personal "hair" trainer—ask lots of questions and don't leave until you get it. You could even bring a flip camera or use the recorder app on your smartphone to capture important bits of styling information.

THE NEW YORK MODEL OFF-DUTY (MOD) CUT

by Harry Josh

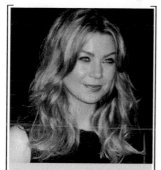

Harry's MOD cut and styling on Ellen Pompeo.

Harry's famous haircut, best for thin to medium straight or wavy hair, almost does the styling for you! The subtle layering lifts hair to bring out natural waves in a fresh, edgy way. It's a layered cut to give you that nonchalant "I just woke up with great hair" look of the world's top supermodels.

1. HAVE YOUR STYLIST trim along the perimeter of your cut to establish the length. If your hair is healthy, he can use a razor to get a "shattered" hipster effect on the ends.

2. IN THE FRONT, the stylist should frame your face with the shortest pieces, beginning at the bottom of the chin.

3. THE FINAL STEP: Layers, just enough but not too many. They should be longer than the front pieces to keep the cut from looking like a shag. You can layer a bit more in the front than in the back to keep the back looking thick.

TO STYLE Your stylist can blow your look straight or with a natural wave using a brush and blow-dryer. At home Harry says to just spritz in a little dry hair texturizer before or after air-drying.

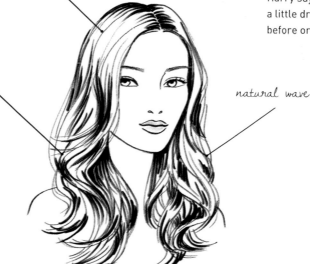

slightly shorter front pieces

light layers

natural wave

BOOK AN APPOINTMENT WITH...

OSCAR BLANDI
The Italian Hair Stallion

Sexy but subtle is the way Oscar Blandi likes hair to look, and his star clients (Kelly Ripa, Sofia Vergara, Rosario Dawson, Jessica Alba, Faith Hill) are great models of his work. His Madison Avenue salon is also a go-to destination for countless young socialites who want to buy into the concept of hair that looks rich but still real, simple but super sexy. Oscar's Italianized English, a remnant from his childhood in Naples, is also pretty sexy, and when he speaks and touches your hair, you feel instantly more glam.

"My personal style and the cut I tend to gravitate toward is a soft, natural style that looks very 'wash and wear.' I like women to look sexy, but in a subtle way."

—Oscar Blandi

Oscar's Cheap Trick
For super-moisturized locks, Oscar says, "Your daily conditioner can double as a treatment by applying to dry hair and leaving it in for fifteen minutes under a shower cap." When you rinse, your hair will feel luxuriously soft and have great shine.

THE GLAMOROUS CUT FOR CURLS

by Oscar Blandi

This is the cut that rich girls and actresses known for their curls, like Oscar's client Julianna Margulies, get so they can wear their hair naturally curly.

1. ASK YOUR STYLIST to help determine the length he's going to cut the front and the back. Blandi thinks right below the collarbone in the back and slightly shorter in the front is the chicest length for this cut, but because curls spring up when dry, he suggests having your stylist cut your hair about two inches below the collarbone to compensate for shrinkage.

2. CUT BANGS right below cheekbones (they, too, will spring up).

3. TO FRAME THE SIDES, your stylist should slide the scissors diagonally downward from the end of your bangs down the length of your hair on each side.

4. CUT LAYERS into the sides, section by section, being sure none of the layers are more than an inch and a half shorter than the overall length of that particular section. This assures you won't get the dreaded "triangle effect" so common with curly haircuts.

TO STYLE

Your stylist should use a frizz serum or hair oil and diffuser, but at home your hair is wash and wear . . . apply product and air-dry.

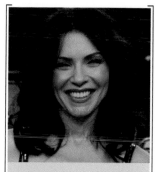

Julianna Margulies works Oscar's cut on the red carpet.

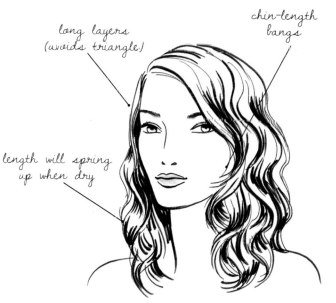

long layers (avoids triangle)

chin-length bangs

length will spring up when dry

Shampoo: How Much Do You Really Need to Spend?

I ride both sides of the fence here. For me, using an expensive shampoo is a little luxury I can't give up. I like the feeling of the rich lather, the delicious fragrance, and the afterglow of silky tresses. Maybe it's because I have three kids, I work, and my time in the shower is sacred to me. I'm partial to Frédéric Fekkai, Morrocanoil, Nexxus Dualiste (some might think I bathe in the stuff I go through it so quickly), L'Oréal Paris Série Professionnel (especially their Série Nature eco-friendly line), and the Aveda Invati hair-thickening line, always sticking to products that are for color-treated hair. David Babaii agrees with me: "It's that small thing you can do for yourself that feels really luxurious; like wearing Chanel perfume when you can't afford a Chanel suit, it gives you a psychological lift." At the same time, I like to alternate in some less expensive brands I've found give the same luxe look and feel, both in the shower and when I'm done styling my hair, such as John Frieda (especially the Sheer Blonde line), Alba Botanica, and Kiss My Face shampoos and conditioners.

I think it's important to mention that I've tried just as many expensive duds that made my hair too greasy or too soft or too smelly as I have inexpensive ones. The bottom line? To find a shampoo that not only makes your hair look great but also makes you feel great may take some experimenting. Mini bottles meant for travel are perfect for this. What to do with the full-bottle busts you buy along the way? Don't throw them (and your money) down the drain, or let those bottles sit unused, taking up space in the shower. Use them on your child, dog, or recycle them as body conditioner. Just apply to arms, legs, and torso after cleansing and rinse off—it'll make your skin silky, and you won't need to moisturize when you get out.

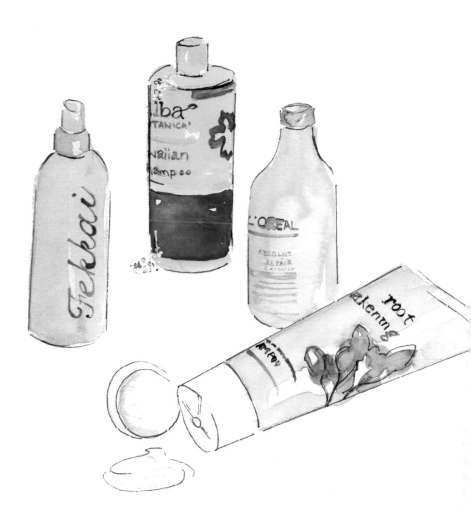

*Using an expensive shampoo is
a little luxury I can't give up....
At the same time, I like to alternate
in some less expensive brands
I've found give the same luxe
look and feel.*

Get Professional Results: Your Hair Tool Kit at Any Price

Wondering where to spend and where to save when it comes to your hair tools? Here's what you need and what you don't.

HEAT APPLIANCES

In general, spending some money on your heat tools will pay off in less heat damage and healthier, more expensive-looking hair. Better tools will also save you time because they work more efficiently and, at least in my book, time is money.

THE BLOW-DRYER

Worth an investment, a high-tech blow-dryer can even cut drying time in half, saving your hair from excess heat (and your arm from all that lifting!). Though you don't need a $200-plus one like a pro does, the $8.99 old-fashioned Big Bird kind won't do it, either. Look for something middle of the road or better that takes advantage of new technology with heat output of 1800 watts or more. Be sure it has a separate attachment nozzle for directing heat more specifically. Tourmaline dryers distribute heat most evenly without disrupting the cuticle and causing frizz.

SAVE

Conair YOU Reel 2-in-1 Styler, $34.99; Goody Heat Flash Dry Blow Dryer, $36.99

SPLURGE

Solano 3300 XtraLite Dryer, $159 at Ulta.com; T3 Featherweight Professional Hair Dryer, $200

CURLING IRONS

Most stylists have a few different irons in different sizes, but if you can't afford a large barrel (two-inch diameter) for looser curls and a small diameter (half-inch diameter) for tighter ones, go for the large barrel—the curls it creates are the most forgiving and if you run it down the length of hair before you curl it to flatten the cuticle, it can double as a straightening iron.

SAVE

Remington T-Studio Ceramic Pearl Professional Styling Wand, $29.99

SPLURGE

Sultra The Bombshell One-Inch Rod Curling Iron, $130

THE STRAIGHTENING IRON

I'm addicted to mine. When I'm short on time and need a polished look pronto, it's the straightening iron I plug in. You can even learn to easily curl your hair with it. Choose one with a ceramic coating to help distribute heat evenly; these get super hot super fast but won't scorch your hair.

SAVE

Remington T-Studio Pearl Ceramic Wide Straightener, $39.99

SPLURGE

Solano SleekHeat450 Flat Iron, $159.95 at Ulta.com

BRUSHES

Got a drawer full of brushes? Toss 'em! These are the only three you'll ever need.

THE PADDLE BRUSH

A flat brush that every stylist swears by for detangling and blow-drying hair 75 percent dry before styling with the medium round brush. It can be a combination of natural and nylon bristles, but stay away from metal bristles that tend to tear your hair.

SAVE

Conair Mega Ceramic Paddle Brush, $8.99,
Ricky's Classic Black Boar & Porcupine Paddle, $9.99;
Goody QuikStyle Paddle Brush, $11.99 (with microfiber to pull the water out and quicken dry time)

SPLURGE

Aveda Wooden Paddle Brush, $20

THE ROUND BRUSH

The most important tool for achieving a great result with a blow-dry. Stylists usually have a slew of different sizes, but as Adir Abergel told me, "Honestly, I only use the medium-size one." So there you have it. Get yourself one good-quality medium-size round brush (two-and-a-half-inch diameter) with natural boar bristles. You can often find the professional brands online or at a beauty supply store—and they're often less expensive than some fancy boutique brand brushes.

SAVE

Remington Frizz Therapy Round Brush, $9.99

SPLURGE

Ibiza Hair EX3 Medium Brush, $44 (Adir loves it); Boar-bristle Marilyn brushes (Harry Josh swears by them); Flatter Me Too 2½˝, $32; Jeli Ceramica 2½˝, $34

THE MASON PEARSON BRUSH

Some pros say it has to be the real thing, but others say it's the combination of closely placed natural bristles mixed with nylon ones that makes this brush so special, not the brand itself. Use this kind of brush for smoothing and brushing hair out at the end of a blow-dry and throughout the day.

SAVE

Denman grooming brushes (with natural bristle and nylon pins), from $9.99 to $15.99; Sonia Kashuk Kashuk Tools Hairbrush, $14.99

SPLURGE

Mason Pearson award-winning Popular Model brush, $170

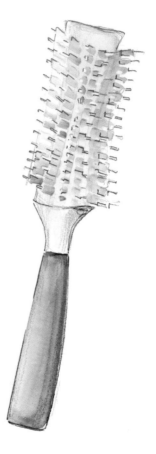

FINE- AND WIDE-TOOTH COMBS

Use a fine-tooth comb for parting and teasing. The secret to teasing without making a tangled or tacky mess, by the way, is to pick up a section of hair half the width of the comb itself. Lift the section into the air, then starting about two inches from the root, begin to compress hair toward the root. I use one of the new wide-tooth combs with argon oil infused into the plastic to neaten and revive a wavy or natural hairstyle without pulling out the curl— while adding shine at the same time (no need for an additional finishing product).

WORTH-IT STYLING PRODUCTS

There are thousands of products to choose from, but I've found that the pros really stick to just a few. Simplifying your choices makes it easier to avoid overdoing it or making the wrong decision. This is an edited list of my favorites. Though not all are inexpensive, they're investments that'll save you from wasting money on products that don't deliver.

THICKENING SPRAY

Spray it on roots and mist it through the length of wet hair to give hair lift and body while keeping it soft and touchable.

MY FAVORITES

Bumble and bumble Thickening Hairspray, $27; Frédéric Fekkai COIFF Bouffant Lifting and Texturizing Spray Gel, $25; göt2b Fat-tastic Thickening Plumping Non-aerosol Hairspray, $5.99

DRY SHAMPOO

A real secret weapon, not just for making dirty hair look clean, but for putting in texture and adding volume. These come in either sprays you hold about ten inches from your scalp and mist into roots, or powders you diffuse in your hands, then rub through your hair. Don't freak out if the dry shampoo makes your hair look white—wait a few minutes till the product dries, then brush through or tousle it in with your fingers and the white disappears.

Baby powder also works as dry shampoo! Socialite Olivia Palermo once told me she carries some around in a ziplock bag—though you need to use it sparingly.

MY FAVORITES

Klorane Gentle Dry Shampoo with Oat Milk, $18;
Oscar Blandi Pronto Dry Shampoo Spray, $21;
Frédéric Fekkai Au Naturel Dry Shampoo, $25

DRY TEXTURIZING SPRAY

Imagine a miracle product that gives you the results of a blow-dryer and curling iron wrapped into one and put in a bottle. That's the genius behind these new hair products. Seriously. They do the work for you. Apply to dry hair, scrunch with your fingers, and it'll look like you had your hair done.

MY FAVORITES

Oribe Dry Texturizing Spray, $39; Redken Wool Shake 08
Gel-Slush Texturizer, $17; John Frieda Luxurious Volume
Anytime Volume Refresher, $6.50

SILICONE DEFRIZZER

Another must-have for curly hair. Modern silicone anti-frizz products are almost weightless and won't make hair feel heavy or greasy. The secret to making them work is to apply from roots to ends when hair is completely wet to lock out humidity from the get-go.

MY FAVORITES

John Frieda Frizz-Ease Original Formula Hair Serum, $9.99;
Citré Shine Shine Miracle Anti-Frizz Serum, $5.99;
Phyto Phytodéfrisant Botanical Hair Relaxing Balm, $26;
Kérastase Nutritive Sérum Oléo-Relax, $39

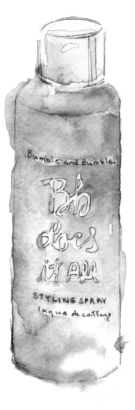

HAIR SPRAY

Look for one that won't leave your hair stiff or helmet-like but keeps the texture moveable and brushable, so you can build style upon style.

MY FAVORITES

Frédéric Fekkai COIFF Sheer Hold Hairspray, $25; Bumble and bumble Does It All Styling Spray, $25; Aveda Air Control Hair Spray, $24; L'Oréal Paris Elnett Satin Hairspray, $14.99; Dove Style+Care Strength & Shine Flexible Hold Hairspray, $3.76

STRAIGHTENING PRODUCTS

Another new-product category, designed to help you get straight and silky hair when you blow-dry at home. These products take out the curl so you don't have to work so hard or kill your hair with heat appliances to get it straight.

MY FAVORITES

Frédéric Fekkai COIFF Contrôle Ironless Straightening Balm, $25; John Frieda Frizz-Ease 3-Day Straight Semi-Permanent Styling Spray, $9.99

CONDITIONING OIL

A newer hair product category, these oils—derived from natural ingredients—condition, defrizz, add texture, and shine, without looking greasy (a contradiction, I know) and are a godsend for curly, coarser hair. For curly, thick, or coarse textures, they can be applied wet to control frizz; for finer hair types, use as a finishing step for shine.

MY FAVORITES

L'Oréal Professionnel Mythic Oil, $29; Moroccanoil Treatment, $40.80; Couture Colour Pequi Oil Treatment, $32; RODIN Olio Lusso by RECINE Luxury Hair Oil, $60; Grapeseed oil from the supermarket—use a tiny bit as a finishing oil for all hair textures.

MUST-HAVE PRO HAIR ACCESSORIES

These are the accessories star stylists use to achieve any of the hairstyles you see on celebrities, and most can be bought at the drugstore.

HAIR CLIPS

You don't wear these in public! But they're key to sectioning strands and clipping up pin curls without making dents.

BOBBY PINS

Your standard bobby pins are used to secure updos. Use them crisscrossed for extra hold. They also make a great hair accessory in their own right: Lots of stars wear visible bobby pins in groupings of two or more to hold back one side of their hair in a classic, chic way. For added style, use Goody hair-colored bobby pins in a shade that matches your hair. Another accessories trick you'll see on many red-carpet hairstyles that's easy to steal: Use bobby pins to attach a piece of jewelry to your hair—it doesn't have to be a treasure from Bulgari or a family heirloom. Try pinning a rhinestone necklace around a bun, a pair of costume jewelry earrings to bedazzle the side of slicked-back hair. Be creative. Be sure to bend one end of the bobby pin so you don't lose the jewel, even if it's not real!

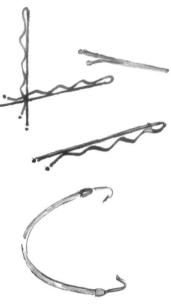

HAIRPINS

These are more-open pins used to secure hair to the bobby-pinned base of an updo and to stick back in any falling-out pieces. A mistake women make is thinking a hairpin will hold a chignon when really the bobby pins do that and the hairpins are the finishing touches for loose strands.

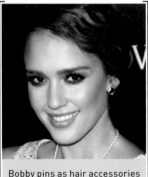

Bobby pins as hair accessories on Jessica Alba

BARRETTES

In gold or silver, these classics from Goody that you may have worn in high school keep reappearing on the fashion runways, even in Milan and Paris. When it comes to hair accessories, simple is always better in my opinion.

HAIR ELASTICS

Pros use bungee elastics, which are sold at beauty supply stores. They let you put a ponytail in place, minus ponytail bumps, and keep it there (it won't slide out or fall down). Like a mini bungee cord, the trick is to secure one end into your hair at the base of where you want to make the ponytail, wrap the cord around and around the hair, and then secure it behind the ponytail (you don't have to match the ends of the clip together).

I also like clear elastic ponytail holders—they always look chic—and rimless hair-color matching elastics from Goody at the drugstore.

HAIR EXTENSIONS

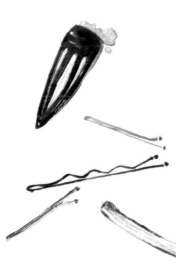

Most pro stylists carry bags of hair with them to give hairstyles thickness, drama, and length, or to fatten up a bun or ponytail. Almost every red-carpet style you see has some extra hair in it, though you'd never know it. They're not the kind of extensions that glue in and damage the hair, though. They clip in just for the night. And there's no reason you can't have a set, too. You can find great ones at beauty supply stores and even at the drugstore; just look for a color that matches your own hair color. Even better, buy blonde human hair extensions with clips online or at a wig store, then take them to your stylist to be custom cut and colored for a one-time investment you'll use again and again. To put them in, all you do is tease a small bit of your real hair in an underneath layer, then secure the clips to the teasing and drop a layer of your unteased hair on top to hide the attachment.

Give Yourself a Pricey Blow-dry
(AND MAKE IT LAST)

THE LONG VERSION

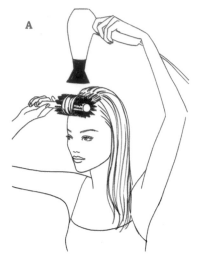

A

You might think of a blow-dry as a style in itself, and this one from Adir Abergel certainly is. But it's more than that. It's also the starting point for just about every red-carpet hairstyle. Think of it like foundation you'd use on your face. It smoothes and shines and acts as a base for any hair look you want to create, be it curly, straight, up, or down. They even do this blow-dry before making a ponytail in Hollywood! I find it übereasy to do myself. But remember, practice makes perfect. As Adir so nicely puts it: "Blow-drying your hair is like riding a bike. It's hard until you figure it out. But the minute it clicks, you'll have fabulous rich hair for the rest of your life." The instructions may seem complicated but once you "get" them, you'll never have to read them again!

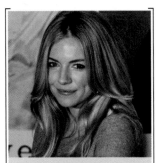

The payoff:
A blow-dry like Sienna Miller's with shine and body

1. GRAB THE BOUNTY!
Instead of a towel out of the shower, Adir uses paper towels to blot out as much moisture as possible without roughing up the hair (friction equals frizz!). Then blow-dry using medium heat, with hair flipped over your head, raking your hand through it like a brush. Stop when hair is still about 50 percent wet. You can also just air-dry to this stage. The idea is to get as much moisture out of the hair without causing frizz or excess heat damage.

2. ADD THICKENING SPRAY to the roots only. It'll give your style grip to hold on to, and because you're not applying it all over, hair texture will remain soft and touchable. Blitz the roots with the blow-dryer, lifting hair with your fingers until hair is 75 percent dry (just slightly damp).

3. SWITCH TO A MEDIUM-SIZE ROUND BRUSH, using high heat and a nozzle on the dryer. Start on the important front sections (by the time you get to the back, you're tired, so put your energy where it matters). Take a section of hair about the width of your brush, comb through it and blow-dry to detangle, smooth, and dry completely; then pull the section in front of your face and roll it back on the brush, wrapping hair toward your face as you blow-dry. Point the nozzle downward (avoids frizz), as in sketch A. You've essentially turned the brush into a heated Velcro roller.

4. DON'T UNWRAP THE BRUSH UNTIL THE SECTION COOLS (at least 20 seconds). If you have time, immediately recoil the curl around your finger, as

in sketch B, and pin it up to set the curl, almost as if it was still wrapped around the brush. (I skip this step on busy mornings.)

5. REPEAT ON ANOTHER FRONT SECTION, then do two giant sections on each side. Remember to grab the top layer of hair, brush through to detangle, and blow-dry to smooth and dry before wrapping the section around the brush and blow-drying it again.

6. NOW'S THE TRICKY PART: the back. Adir says what's important here is to make the ends look beautiful, so don't worry about the part of your hair you can't reach.

Take a section and repeat the smooth, dry, curl, dry, and coil routine on the last few inches of the hair you can reach, as in sketch C. Repeat on rest of the back (you can probably get away with two sections).

7. TAKE OUT THE PINNED CURLS and finger your hair into place. For more smoothness, brush with a Mason Pearson–style brush. Voilà! Chic, shiny, healthy, expensive looking hair! ▶

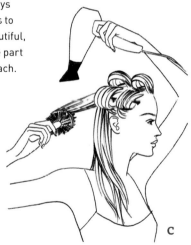

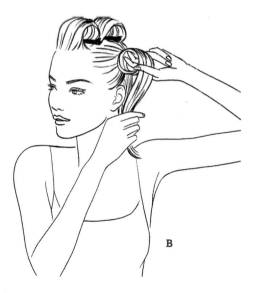

B

C

THE SHORT VERSION

1. Blow-dry on medium heat using your fingers as a brush until hair is just slightly damp.

2. Apply thickening spray to roots and blow-dry them while lifting them up.

3. Use a round brush and high heat on face-framing sections

(over-directing hair in front of your face), as in sketch A.

4. Let each section cool twenty seconds before taking out the brush. This step is key.

5. If you have time, recoil and pin up the curl to let it set, as in sketch B.

6. Repeat with giant sections on each side; when you get to the back, roll just as far as you can reach, as in sketch C.

7. Remove clips and finger your hair into place.

How to Make a Blow-dry Last

Whether you DIY your blow-dry or get one at the salon, here's how to make it look good for more than just the day:

- **Wrap your hair in a towel** instead of a shower cap when you shower. The shower cap lets steam under, which will make hair frizz and lose its smoothness. Of course don't put your head under the shower!

- **Sleep on a silky pillowcase** or wrap your hair in a silk scarf like model Chanel Iman told me she does.

- **Use dry shampoo** as needed to sop up oils at the roots.

- **Flip hair upside down** and brush hair from underneath to smooth without taking out the body or style.

- **Make the most of the natural cycle of a blow-dry:** Day 1, smooth. Day 2, still smooth. Day 3, humidity and sleeping on it have put some wave in, so add some more with a large-barrel curling iron or dry texturizing spray. Day 4, pull it into a messy-chic ponytail. Day 5, shampoo!

Adir's Shine Secret

Flatten the cuticle to create shine. When you flatten the cuticle, your hair reflects light and gets a certain kind of richness that you can't get any other way. This sounds like it may call for straight hair, but actually Adir starts off even his curly styles with his famous blow-dry, straightening the hair first (and at the same time flattening the cuticle) to give it shine, then putting more defined curls back in.

The Top Celebrity Hair Myths

1 **Rarely does a stylist start from wet hair** when he creates a celebrity hairstyle. The take away? You don't have to, either. Celebs come to their hairdressers with clean, dry hair, often washed the night before. I find it easier to air-dry my hair and then go in and style from there, adding thickening lotion if I need some lift, dry shampoo if I need body, then using a blow-dryer or straightening iron to create sleek styles or a curling iron to enhance my natural waves. Or I'll let my hair air-dry for day and then style it for night.

2 **When a star or runway model wears curls,** she didn't just use a diffuser. Usually hair was dried straight and sleek to smooth it down and get rid of frizz, and then the curls were put back in. The take away: You can achieve a similar effect by applying frizz-fighting lotion or hair oil, then wrapping your hair tightly in a snail-like bun to sleeken the curl. Once dry, use a curling iron to give the curls more direction if needed.

3 **Not every celebrity has great hair.** What they do have is great spirit. "Own your hair," says Harry Josh. "Even if you just pull it back, if you own it, it can look amazing. I mean, really, what's so great about Kate Moss's hair? It's medium-fine hair, cut to her shoulders. Nothing special. But we love it because we love the image she portrays. Attitude is everything when it comes to hair."

4 **You can often recognize a boob job in Hollywood,** but fake hair? Tougher to catch. Why is Hollywood hair always so full and lush? Stylists tell me with HDTV, you can see right through hair so they almost always have to pump it up with (invisible) extensions.

Master Luxury Curls That Don't Come Cheap

Here's how to get incredibly chic high-end curls and waves. You can achieve these looks on air-dried or natural hair, but remember that celebrity stylists smooth hair out with a great blow-dry to seal the cuticle before putting the curls in, even on naturally curly hair.

Boho Waves

These are trendier waves that almost look loosely crimped. They run horizontally down your hair instead of parallel like the other curls. Part hair down the center or off-center. Using a small straightening iron, start at the top and jiggle the iron back and forth down the length of hair instead of wrapping hair up in it.

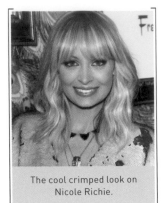

The cool crimped look on Nicole Richie.

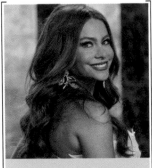

Sofia Vergara's waves are as voluptuous as her body.

Bombshell Waves

This is the super-sexy look. Part hair in the middle or slightly off-center, then begin to curl hair, pointing the iron down to the ground as you curl the hair around the iron without the clip, moving from roots to ends as you wrap the hair. Leave the ends out as you curl, always wrapping hair away from the face.

Uptown/Downtown Waves

Think Blake Lively's famous *Gossip Girl* waves. (I told you how lucrative they were for her . . . Chanel came calling, after all!) Plug in both a curling iron and a straightening iron. Curl large two-inch sections with a curling iron. Once hair is curled, pull out a random curl and straighten it with the straightening iron. The ratio of curls to straight pieces should be about four to one to achieve the ideal mix of uptown glamour and downtown edginess.

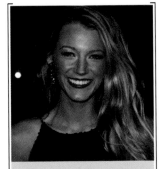

Mix curls and straight strands to get Blake Lively's waves.

Forties Movie Star Waves

This is the modern take on the more structured, retro Veronica Lake (or Jessica Rabbit!) look: Take horizontal sections, this time starting at the roots, bring the iron straight down to the ends (for a straightening iron kind of effect) before curling it back up to the roots. Curl each curl in the same direction. Then make a deep side part, run a smoothing brush (such as Mason Pearson) over hair and tuck one side behind your ear.

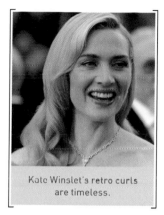

Kate Winslet's retro curls are timeless.

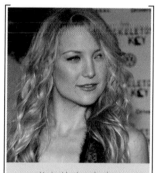

Kate Hudson's the queen of beach waves.

Beach Waves

This is the natural, Kate Hudson look. You may be able to get these curls just by adding a beach spray or dry texturizing lotion to create messy waves and movement. If you need to add more, curl a few scattered horizontal sections of hair, two to four inches wide, throughout your head. Starting at the roots with the clamp of the iron closed (in other words, no hair should be secured in the clamp), wind the section of hair around the curling iron. You'll get a tighter curl at the top and looser curls at the ends.

Red-Carpet Modern Curls

These are more refined glamour curls, the kind you'd wear with a Marchesa gown. Use a small curling iron (quarter- to one-inch diameter) to curl hair section by section, switching direction of the curl each time. One section you roll forward, the next you roll backward. This creates a finger-wave effect that looks natural but very glam. To intensify the ringlets, twist hair like a rope before you curl it.

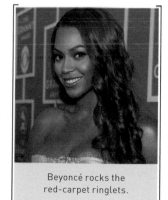

Beyoncé rocks the red-carpet ringlets.

Four Chic Ponytails That Will Make You Look Luxe

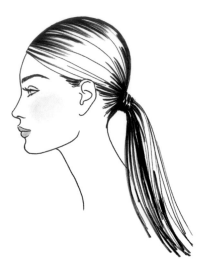

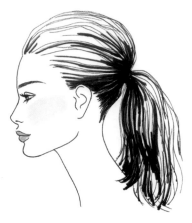

The sleek and sophisticated pony

Pull hair back sleek and low and secure with an elastic or hair bungee cord. Grab a section from the side of the ponytail about one inch thick, run a straightening iron over it, then wrap it around the base of the ponytail to hide the elastic. Use a bobby pin to secure it to the base of the ponytail. Add a decorative pin for night. Chic.

The cheekbone-chiseling ponytail

Tease the crown by using a fine-tooth comb to compress hair down at the root, then pull front sections straight back right over the teased sections and use a bungee elastic so as not to crush the volume. Or spritz hair with a dry texturizing spray first to add the texture without teasing, let dry, then pull hair gently back. You can also spray just the tail for bedheadlike volume.

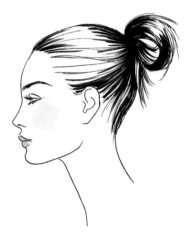

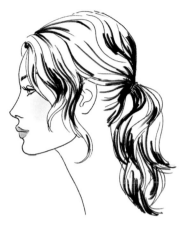

The casual and chic pony-bun

The boho curly ponytail

Pull elastic around hair once and on the second time around, pull hair only half through to create a messy-looking bunlike effect. You can wrap the end of the tail around the bun and secure it with bobby pins for a slightly more "done" look.

Curl hair according to one of the instructions in the Master Luxury Curls section, then twist and secure hair in a bungee elastic, letting whatever falls in the front fall where it lands, preferably in front of one of your eyes.

MY EASY GO-TO UPDO

This is the perfect look to put together when you have a crazy-busy day but only five minutes for your hair.

1. Gather your hair in your hands in a high ponytail. Without securing the tail in an elastic, begin twisting your hair until it coils and begins to wrap around itself into a bun.

2. Secure bun. Mine holds with just an elastic, but if you need more support, add a few hairpins. Goody Simple Styles Spin Pins, which work like a screw by anchoring your hair in place, are another great option.

Couturize Your Haircut & Style

PARK AVENUE PRETTY

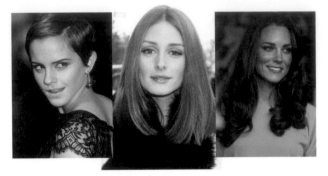

If your hair is short, try a sleek pixie. Style straight and chic with lots of shine. **Think:** *Emma Watson, Kelly Ripa*

If your hair is shoulder-length, go for layers just at the bottom and add chin-length face-framing pieces. Wear it straight and sleek to catch the light. **Think:** *Olivia Palermo, Pippa Middleton*

If your hair is long, keep it simple, layering just on the ends. Wear it straight with volume at the roots or beautifully curled. **Think:** *Kate Middleton, Anne Hathaway*

HOLLYWOOD BOHO

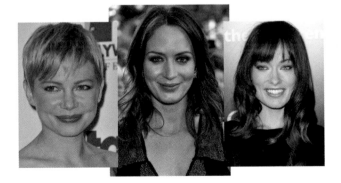

If your hair is short, try a slightly asymmetrical pixie. Air-dry for a messy-chic effect. **Think:** *Michelle Williams, Alexa Chung*

If your hair is shoulder-length, get a cut with long layers. Air-dry or use a dry texturizing spray to mess it up and add natural wave. **Think:** *Emily Blunt, Nicole Richie*

If your hair is long, get a layered haircut with long bangs for a boho vibe. Style with a dry texturizing spray to add a cool factor, whether you wear it down or pulled back into a teased and textured ponytail. **Think:** *Olivia Wilde, Zooey Deschanel*

GLAM GLOBE-TROTTER

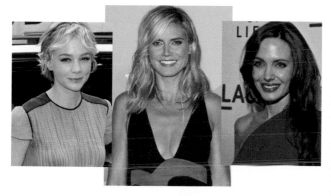

If your hair is short, go for a short but not-so-precise bob with long fringy bangs or a fuss-free pixie. Air-dry for everyday, but add some curls to glam it up for night. **Think:** *Carey Mulligan, Halle Berry*

If your hair is shoulder-length, get a long-layered, low-maintenance cut. Wear it down and natural, or all pulled back into a low ponytail or messy knot. **Think:** *Heidi Klum, Sienna Miller*

If your hair is long, have just the ends gently layered to give hair body even when you do nothing. To style? Just brush! Or add volume at the roots and blow-dry off your face, even partless. **Think:** *Angelina Jolie, Julianne Moore*

MODERN MOVIE STAR

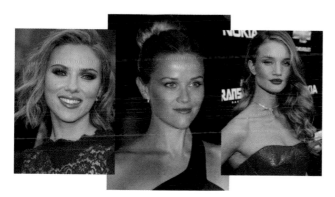

If your hair is short, try a long bob. Wear it smooth and shiny or sensuously curled. At night, add a fun beaded headband. **Think:** *Scarlett Johansson, Charlize Theron*

If your hair is shoulder-length, get minimal layering, which is better for adapting to different hair "roles." Wear it parted to the side, straight and shiny to catch the light on the red carpet, or pulled back into a chic chignon. **Think:** *Reese Witherspoon, January Jones*

If your hair is long, get a simple cut, minimal layering, shorter pieces around the face but no bangs. Wear it parted to the side with dramatic curls, Veronica Lake style. **Think:** *Rosie Huntington-Whiteley, Megan Fox, Kim Kardashian*

THE UPDO THAT'S CLASSY INSTEAD OF TRASHY

A sexy chignon is one way to make your hair look enviably wealthy instantaneously. "Every woman looks more regal with hair off her face, especially if you show your neck and pile your hair to make height at the crown. It makes your neck look longer, your cheekbones higher, your whole persona seem more expensive. It's not even a question that I'm going to try an updo with an Oscar gown," says Creighton. Whether you make a topknot, a low ballerina bun, or just nonchalantly pull hair back into a messy bun, I say wear it with your business clothes (to look promotable) or with an LBD to look like an heiress (or should I say hair-ess?). The trick to make the chignon look effortless is to keep some natural texture so it doesn't look stuffy, to not overspray it, and to keep some wispy pieces around the face or a little height at the roots for a more face-flattering effect. If your updo feels too fancy or done, go low-key with either your makeup or your outfit—make your red lipstick look more lived-in by applying it with a finger, or pull on a leather or denim jacket to tone down your gown.

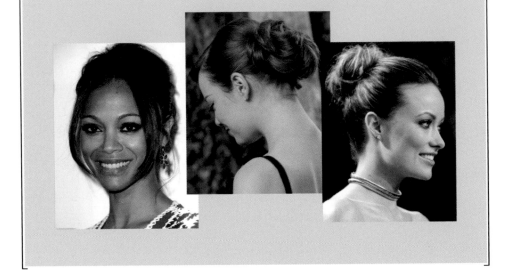

Now you have the tools and tips…

to upgrade your haircut and style to create your own luxe look. I've explained how closely hair and self-esteem are related, and I hope you'll take me seriously when I tell you that spending time and effort on your hair is well worth it. You'll reap the benefits, big-time, and feel happier, more confident, and more in control of your life. Plus, these techniques become second nature after a few goes at it, just like riding a bike. So before we move on to hair color, another key component to expensive-looking hair, let's review what makes your hair look chic . . . and what makes it look cheap.

HAIR THAT MAKES YOU LOOK LIKE

You Don't Have a Dime

- Unruly frizz
  (Where's the shine?)

- Too much teasing
  (Think Snooki.)

- Split ends, yikes!

- Too many layers

- Product OD (hair looks hard or greasy)

- Greasy roots

HAIR THAT MAKES YOU LOOK LIKE

A Million Bucks

- Diamond sparkle
  (hair reflects light)

- Silky texture

- Looks amazing but effortless

- Curls or waves that have some definition, no frizz!

- Lots of body . . . in all the right places (too much on the top looks too done and old-fashioned)

- Touchable!

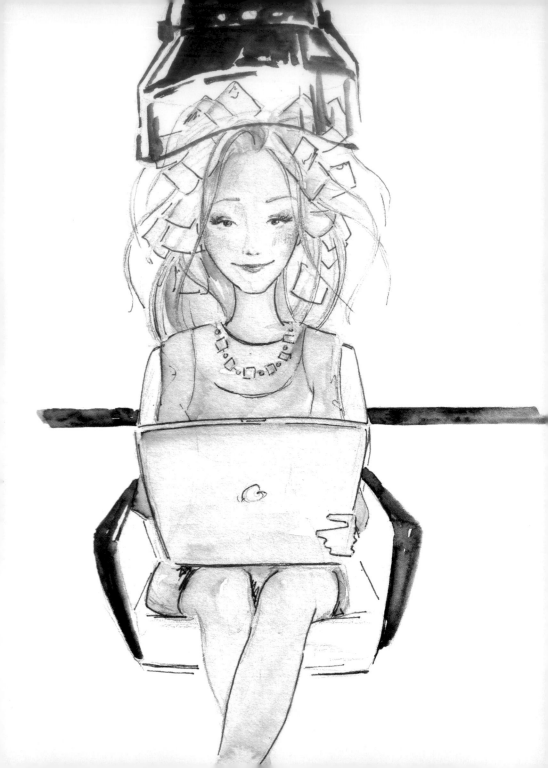

2

The Hair Color of Money

—— Rich-Girl Highlights without a Trust Fund ——

Rich girls always have that perfect set of highlights color that you know has to be chemically enhanced (because who has such blondeness naturally after age ten?) but looks completely natural and believable, not phony or fake. What's that all about? In my *Glamour* column, I've often half-jokingly referred to blonde hair as gold-card-colored hair, referencing the Amex card color you potentially need to get and maintain golden, Blake Lively–esque tresses (not too yellow, not too honey, not too white). But it's not just the gold-card-colored blondes in Hollywood or even the lighter, brighter platinum-card blondes like Kate Hudson who spend the big bucks on hair color. Brunettes and redheads are in on the action, too. I'll go so far as to say there's not one brunette or redhead you've seen on-screen or on the red carpet who doesn't have a high-end dye job going on. Hair color is *the* secret ingredient that gives hair richness on TV, in the movies, and, most relevant to you and me, in real life. So how can you get this kind of color without a sugar daddy or mortgaging your house?

The Seven Qualities of Expensive-Looking Hair Color

Money spent on your hair color can have a *huge* return on investment. But that's when it's done right, so it's important to know the qualities of good hair color. I'll get into them more specifically shade by shade, but here are seven basic tenets all hair colors should meet to look luxe.

1 **Expensive color looks natural.** Rich hair color looks real, believable, like it could be the color you were born with. It's color that looks like it could be growing out of your own head without a hair colorist's intervention.

2 **Say no to "shoe polish" color.** Color that looks the most expensive contains lots of different shades blended together for a multidimensional effect that you'd only notice if you looked very closely. It's not a solid one-color mass.

3 **Luxe color is a mixture of highlights and lowlights.** That's colorist speak for a mix of different shades woven together so that none of them stand out individually, yet you can tell that some strands are lighter, others darker. The contrasting tones add depth to keep the color from washing out your skin tone.

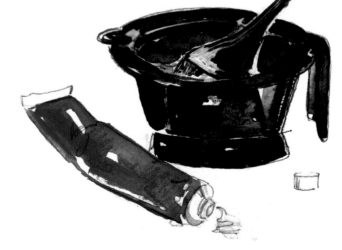

4 **Expensive-looking color has strategically placed brighter strands around the face and is darker in the back.** This mimics natural hair color patterns (even natural blondes have darker hair around the nape).

5 **Hair color that looks the richest doesn't veer too far away from a woman's virgin hair color.** The rule of thumb is three shades max in either direction. This respects that Mother Nature knew what she was doing and is designed to enhance what you start with instead of stripping it away.

6 **Healthy shine is just as important as color.** For color to look rich, it needs to have a glossy, shiny finish to give it a three-dimensional effect.

7 **Finally, expensive-looking color doesn't look too perfect.** It's not totally uniform in tone or placement, because perfect hair color looks as unbelievably phony as a bad nose job. Mother Nature doesn't even do perfect; a good colorist knows better than to try.

The Biggest Hair Color Mistake Women Make?

Going for flashy instead of classy! Let me use what I like to call the Ferrari theory of beauty consumerism, the miscued belief that the more you pay, the more showy your results should be. You paid for the Ferrari (loud, in-your-face), so why did you get an Audi (quietly luxe)? Why are your highlights understated, subtle, and elegant when you paid for bold, brash, and in-your-face? A good colorist will steer you in the classier direction of understated elegance and quietly try to explain why (remember when I told you taste doesn't come with a Platinum Card?), but some women still don't get the difference. Smart girls know that you don't have to see the money you spent to get your money's worth!

Color-by-Color: How to Get Expensive Blonde, Brunette, or Red Hair

The ideas in this section are meant to inspire you to upgrade your hair color and get your chicest, most luxurious shade. You can take these suggestions to your colorist or give them a spin yourself with the DIY tips that you'll find on pages 58–59.

Making Your Blonde Hair Look Expensive

In general, blonde is the priciest hair color there is because it requires the most frequent, expensive upkeep. But there are also some ways to look and feel like a blonde without paying the price.

The Most High-End, High-Maintenance, Expensive Blonde

The buttery or baby blonde look you see on stars like Gwyneth Paltrow, Blake Lively, and Kate Hudson is going to cost you. To get this superlight effect, you need to have the base of your hair lightened to a light blonde (more golden if you want the Gwyneth/Blake look or more platinum if you want the Kate look), then have highlights put on top of the newly lightened hue to make it even lighter and to add that multidimensional sparkle. That's two processes, and you'll pay for each one. And if your hair is dark and won't go light in one step, you'll have to do the lightening part twice—and pay for it twice—on top of the highlights. So skip this look if you're not a light brunette capable of getting blonde in one step, unless you enjoy practically living in a colorist's chair and whipping out your credit card, because that's what it'll take to maintain it . . . every two weeks. Plus, because it's such a stretch from your own natural look, it'll be expensive, but it won't look expensive (reread the seven qualities of expensive-looking hair section if you don't believe me).

HIGHLIGHTS: PINSTRIPES OR CHUNKS?

There are two ways to go with highlights, and though the thinner ones look richer in general because they're more subtle and blend in, they do take a skillful application and natural approach or they can look just as striped as chunks. Chunks on the other hand, are a great way to get a lot of bright for your buck. A blondish piece on each side of your face may be all you need to feel blonde, but avoid the roots so chunks don't look too obvious as they grow out.

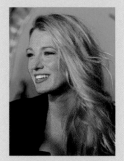

Pinstripes

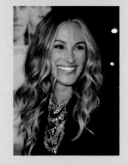

Chunks

Go Blonde for Less

If I haven't scared you away from going blonde, you can make it more affordable. Here are a few ways to pull it off without going broke.

- **You don't have to do the highlights every appointment.** If you're a double-process superlight blonde or covering gray, by keeping up with the roots via the base-lightening step every two or three weeks, you can stretch out the more expensive highlight appointments to every three or four color sessions (that's nine to twelve weeks). It still won't be cheap, but it will cost less, a lot less, than it does for Blake and Gwyneth.

- **Not up for that kind of expenditure or maintenance?** You can get a blonde effect like Sarah Jessica Parker, Jennifer Aniston, or yours truly, with highlights on your own dark base every two or three months (some women can stretch it out to six!). The highlights give you the feeling of blonde, especially if you ask that they be concentrated around the face. Your own natural base color becomes the lowlights, which helps camouflage roots because they blend in with your base as they grow out.

- **To get away with even fewer appointments,** go in about every six weeks and have your colorist paint the hair line or bump the base—both techniques take just a few minutes (though you'll have to dry your wet hair) and many salons will comp the touch-up for regular clients. Do this once or twice between highlights and you'll be able to stretch them to every four or even six months.

- **Another way to get this look for less** is to ask for a half-head or just face-framing highlights. Natural color is darker in the back than the front anyway, so why pay for it? For how to highlight your hair yourself, see page 59.

- **Perhaps the most low-cost, low-maintenance way to add some blondness:** Get a golden gloss on your light brown or dirty blonde hair, or try a semipermanent home color kit a shade or two lighter than your hair color. The former will add golden shimmer and shine that'll brighten up your face with no regrowth; the latter will lighten up your base a smidge but fade away without roots.

Making Your Brown Hair Look Expensive

Brunettes have lots of choices, depending on how dark they are to start. If you're a light brown and you want to go blonde, you can use any of the methods mentioned earlier. If you're a medium brown, you may be able to get away with blonding, or you can go for very subtle highlights a shade or two lighter than your own (ask your colorist to use a tint instead of a bleach, and golden colors like chestnut, sandy brown, or light coconut, avoiding reds and coppers). Highlights on brunettes should be so thin they're almost invisible, so they add dimension and reflect light without changing your hair color.

Highlights on brunettes should be so thin they're almost invisible, so they add dimension and reflect light without changing your hair color.

BEST HAIR COLOR BANG FOR YOUR BUCK

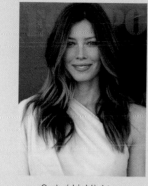

Ombré highlights on
Jessica Biel

Best highlighting technique if you can't afford highlights: Ombré coloring. Tips are lighter and the color fades discreetly up the hair shaft, giving you brightness and the feeling of blondness without the root headache.

Cheapest color to maintain: It's a tie. Both brunettes and redheads can get away with just a clear or colored gloss for shine, inexpensive at the salon and easy to do at home.

Most expensive color to maintain: Platinum/white. Not pretty, not natural, and not cheap. But it looks cheap, except on Gwen Stefani, who can get away with it. Need I say more?

Cheapest root fix: Another tie. Curls camouflage demarcation lines. Changing your part also works—brush hair back, zigzag it, or wear a partless ponytail.

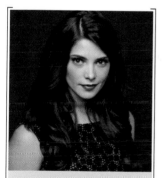

Ashley Greene's brunette
hair with a mink gloss effect

Expensive Brunette for Less

- **Ask for a warm gloss.** Medium brunettes looking for a less expensive way to take the edge off can minimize ashiness with a warm gloss, or deepen their hair out of the mousy spectrum by going a shade or two darker for a deeper, richer effect. At the salon, ask for shades like cocoa, mink, and coffee.

- **Try ombré highlights.** Another option for medium to dark brown hair is ombré highlights, which start at the ends instead of the roots and fade out midway up the hair shaft. Ask your colorist to keep the bleach strongest on the tips and less opaque as it moves upward to give you that gradual fade-out effect.

- **If your hair is raven, almost black:** You can lighten it a shade or two to take the edge off at the salon or at home (try a dark chocolate hue), or embrace your deep, sultry hue like Kim Kardashian and just apply a clear gloss to bring out the shine.

Luxurious Color for Redheads

If you're a natural redhead, your hair will look richest if you enhance it instead of trying to change it. Highlights can wash you out or make you look like a multicolored corn on the cob.

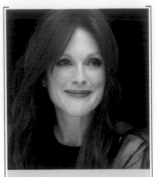

Julianne Moore's hair always looks rich and natural.

- **One way to get around this is to do lowlights.** Adding darker shades of red will make your own hair color the highlight color.

- **Or stick with a solid allover red.** Either match it to your own red with a permanent, semipermanent, or gloss; take it richer and brighter with a solid fiery tone (think Christina Hendricks); or go deeper, darker, more auburn, or nature-based (think Julianne Moore). When you notice the color fading, repeat (reds fade faster than brunettes or blondes).

Adding darker shades of red will make your own hair color the highlight color.

My Hair Colorist BFFs Share Their Philosophy and Advice

BOOK AN APPOINTMENT WITH...

SHARON DORRAM

The Highlight Queen

Sharon Dorram is the go-to girl for celebrity and society blondes in New York. Her clients have run the gamut from Nicole Kidman (who she colored in the star's bathroom) to Tory Burch. What defines her look is the placement and use of lowlights, which are the base-color strands she doesn't put in the foils, that help give hair that sexy, sun-streaked, übernatural look as well as the golden gloss she applies at the end to blend it altogether and add shine. The result? Beautiful color with a kick that is enviably elegant.

Sharon is all about making your hair color look as it might have when you were a child at the beach all summer: sun-streaked but strategically so to best accentuate your features in an individualized, personalized, "couture" way that reads elegant and chic.

Sharon's Pet Peeve

Highlights without any lowlights. Some women come in with hair that looks more like a single process than highlights because there's no depth left. She'll use a tint that matches your roots to put back in the darkness and bring back the beauty and richness.

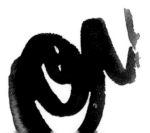

BOOK AN APPOINTMENT WITH...

DOUG MACINTOSH
The Jersey Boy Making It in the Big City

Art school dropout Doug Macintosh began his hair color existence in a New Jersey salon, where his boss told him he was wasting his time and talent and needed to hightail it to the big city. That he did, apprenticing for one of the top colorists of the eighties and nineties before setting up shop as color director of Manhattan's John Sahag Workshop, where his high-profile clients include Renée Zellweger, Jennifer Aniston, Catherine Zeta-Jones, Carey Mulligan, and even Hillary Clinton. He specializes in adjusting a client's color to their personality and profession. He's a big talker and a big listener, and by getting to know his clients he's able to meet their hair color needs.

"Subtle Upper East Side highlights work on a lawyer, but not on a funky Web designer, who might be better suited to big streaks or a vibrant single-process color."

—Doug Macintosh

Doug's Pet Peeve

Color that doesn't match your look, lifestyle, or skin tone. Color should look good without makeup, so don't wear any when you get your color done.

Doug's Cheap Trick

Boost your blonde by pouring leftover champagne from a party over your hair and then blow-drying for five minutes for natural-looking sun-kissed highlights.

BOOK AN APPOINTMENT WITH...

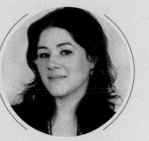

TRACEY CUNNINGHAM

The Hollywood Color Star

Some of the most gorgeous heads of hair in Hollywood—
Cameron Diaz, Gwyneth Paltrow, Jennifer Lopez—get that way
thanks to Tracey Cunningham. A former nanny/chef/assistant to
Bette Midler, Tracey went to beauty school and, after lots of hard work
assisting and manning a blow-dryer (she was dubbed Best Blow-Out Artist
of 1999 by *Allure*), finally got a chance to do color. It's taken her far: She's a
consultant for Redken and heads her own salon.

*Tracey's color tends to veer to the high-
maintenance movie star variety, like the two-
step monthly, buttery blonding look she does on
Gwyneth Paltrow (single process to lighten the
base, with highlights on top).*

Tracey's Pet Peeve

Women who go for a color
without taking the time to
understand the maintenance
from both a time and financial
perspective. "Commit to what
you're prepared to keep up,"
says Tracey, explaining why a
low-maintenance girl shouldn't
try to go Gwyneth blonde.

Tracey's Cheap Trick

A clear gloss. Tracey uses
Redken Shades EQ in her salon
and charges $125, but some salons
offer the service for as low as $30.
"It'll add tons of shine and make
your hair look richer and more
expensive even if you don't color
it," she says. My own supercheap
glossing tip? John Frieda
Luminous Color Glaze Clear
Shine, $9.99 at the drugstore.

Do Your Own Color Like a Celebrity Pro

More and more women are becoming their own hair colorists, and there are a few reasons it makes sense.

With the economy being what it is, salon color isn't even an option for many women.

With the trend toward more subtle hair color that is only a couple of shades lighter or darker than what you start with, doing it yourself becomes more feasible and less of a stretch, even if you have absolutely no idea what you're doing.

There are more and more high-end color kits on the market designed to give you salon-quality color at home, from salon brands like Frédéric Fekkai to upscale but affordable brands like John Frieda.

The technology behind home hair color continues to evolve and many home kits even include tools that mimic those the pros use to help you get better and better results.

These home hair color trends come down to exactly the premise of this book: There's a huge gap between what women want to look like and what they can afford to look like. Luckily, the convergence of these trends, economic realities, and technology are all in sync to help you get your best at-home color ever. Ready to DIY?

TO FIND THE RIGHT BOX, you need to know what color and tone you are starting out with as well as what color and tone you're trying to achieve. Doug Macintosh looks at his clients' eye colors and reads their skin tones to determine whether to go golden or ashy. This is a trick you can steal to find your best home hair dye kit: Go for golden shades if your eyes are brown or hazel and if your skin is sallow to medium-toned. Stick to ashy shades if your eyes are blue or green and

if your skin is pale. Still in doubt? Go golden. It's more forgiving and gives a richer effect anyway.

IF YOU'RE A FIRST-TIMER and have a relationship with a colorist, you can plead poor and ask her to suggest a kit and color to buy that will give you the effect you want. She may even give you some of her base formula to take home. Alternatively, do your research online before you hit the store. All color brands have websites designed to help you narrow in on the right box of color and it's easier to view the shades and compare them to your own on a computer screen than a tiny hair color box. Some sites even let you download your own picture and "try on" a specific color.

CHOOSE A KIT NO MORE THAN TWO SHADES LIGHTER OR DARKER than your own hair so you can't get into too much trouble if you make a mistake.

TRY A NO-DRIP FOAM FORMULA. This newer formulation is less likely to drip in your eyes or end up someplace you don't want it.

ALWAYS BUY TWO BOXES. Women who regularly do their own color tell me there's never enough in one box, especially if their hair is long.

FOLLOW THE DIRECTIONS REALLY CAREFULLY and set a timer so you don't get distracted. It's always better to take the color off early than late.

PAINT HIGHLIGHTS RIGHT ON THE HAIR with a toothbrush instead of wrapping hair up in foils. Called Balayage, this technique used by the pros is actually more goof-proof because the formula will be less concentrated and just on the surface.

HIGHLIGHT from the ends to about midway up the strand, applying less and less color as you move up

so that the roots are almost bare. You'll get the look of highlights with less chance of making a visible mistake, and you won't have any regrowth to worry about.

PLACE THE HIGHLIGHTS like a pro: three on each side framing the face, three along each side of the head, and three at the crown, for a total of fifteen highlights.

For more pro application ideas, check out YouTube, being sure to only copy a professional. (Unless the amateur has really great hair and you see the after, not just the before!)

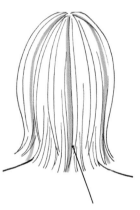

three on each side of your face

three in the back

three on each side of your profile

Get Expensive-Looking Color on the Cheap

- **Be a hair spy.** Investigate women's hair on the bus, in yoga class, or at the office. See a color you like? Ask who did it. Or walk into a chic salon you've spotted and check out the hair color on the employees. Like a look? Ask who did it. It's usually another employee. This can be a great way to discover an up-and-coming colorist with prices that haven't hit the stratosphere yet. You can also now discover up-and-comers on the website StyleSeat.com, which I told you about earlier. It lets real women book a colorist the way a model or magazine editor would—by checking out their portfolio.

- **Spend the money at a top salon to get a few Balayage highlights.** They're painted right on your hair, strategically placed, instead of wrapped in foil. This can last up to six months.

- **Bring visuals of color you like and want to try.** If you forget, grab a magazine and flip through it with your hair colorist during the initial consultation.

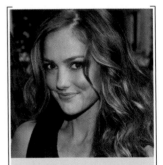

- **See a junior colorist at a high-end salon.** They've probably apprenticed with the star colorist and wouldn't be there if the salon didn't have his or her back. Expect to pay about half as much as for the top salon talent.

- **Ask your stylist to do a finer highlight at the root, getting thicker and chunkier down the length.** This process will avoid a severe root line, something Minka Kelly's colorist, George Papanikolas, does for his clients on a budget.

Minka Kelly's highlights get gradually thicker down the length.

WORK YOUR
Hair Color Budget

IF YOU CAN AFFORD TO GO TO A SALON EVERY SIX MONTHS

Skip single-process color unless you want to try it yourself. Get minimal face-framing highlights on the bottom third of your hair or just on the tips.

IF YOU CAN AFFORD TO GO TO THE SALON EVERY THREE TO FOUR MONTHS

You can get full, half, or face-framing highlights. Ask the colorist to keep the highlights as thin as possible at the root, thickening as they go down to avoid a demarcation line. Keep some of your own darkness in the highlight mix so roots will blend in with the base. When hair starts to look dark, stop by to have the base bumped or the hairline lightened—it'll hold you off another six weeks or so

IF YOU CAN AFFORD TO GO TO THE SALON ONCE A MONTH OR EVEN MORE

You can get single-process coloring or even base coloring and highlights (double process). Basically, try whatever color you want. But beware the time commitment, as well as the financial commitment, before you go this route.

Couturize Your Hair Color

PARK AVENUE PRETTY

If your hair is blonde, get golden highlights with hair line painting and a finishing gloss to blend it all together. Think: *Gwyneth Paltrow, Diane Kruger*

If you're a brunette, go for subtle highlights a shade or two lighter than your hair, just around the face, with a gloss slightly deeper than your own hair on top. Think: *Chanel Iman, Kate Middleton*

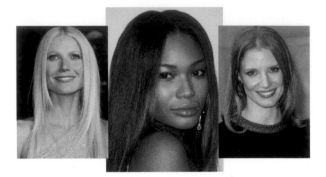

If you're a redhead, try a light golden copper gloss or honey-toned highlights. Think: *Jessica Chastain, Marcia Cross*

HOLLYWOOD BOHO

If your hair is blonde, let your roots grow out for a more lived-in, less perfect look. Think: *Carey Mulligan, Nicole Richie*

If you're a brunette, lighten up the ends and a few select pieces around your face for a sultry, sun-kissed glow. Think: *Rachel Bilson, Leighton Meester*

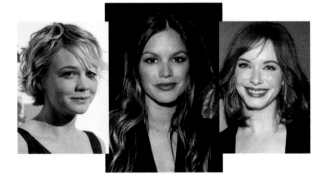

If you're a redhead, go bold and fiery, even a little artificial. Think: *Christina Hendricks, Rihanna*

GLAM GLOBE-TROTTER

If your hair is blonde, go for a dirty blonde with lots of low-lights so roots won't show when you can't get to the colorist. **Think:** *Gisele Bündchen, Kate Moss*

If you're a brunette, enhance your own hue with a hair-matching or auburn gloss to add subtle brightness and shine. **Think:** *Freida Pinto, Milla Jovovich*

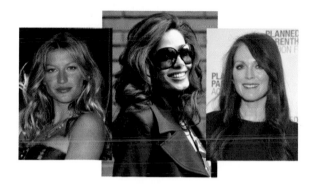

If you're a redhead, go for a shimmering strawberry base that matches your skin tone, with a few lighter pieces around the front. **Think:** *Julianne Moore, Isla Fisher*

MODERN MOVIE STAR

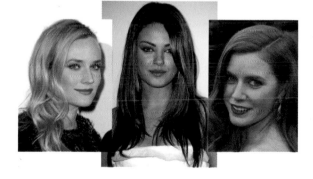

If your hair is blonde, go rich and buttery with a lightened base and gold or baby blonde highlights. **Think:** *Diane Kruger, Reese Witherspoon*

If you're a brunette, stay deep and glossy with a few face-brightening highlights. **Think:** *Mila Kunis, Megan Fox*

If you're a redhead, brighten up your natural color and add a glossy shine. **Think:** *Amy Adams, Emma Stone*

How to Maintain Your Hair Color Investment

So once you've got your color where you want it, how do you keep it that way? It's all about protecting your investment! Here's how:

- **Wait forty-eight hours after fresh color before washing it.** I can't find any studies that prove this works, but it's something a colorist once told me and I've always done it, figuring it certainly can't hurt!

- **Keep it dirty.** I'm only sort of kidding. The less often you wash, the less your color will fade. Use dry shampoo to sop up greasy roots between shampoos.

- **Use high-tech anti-color faders.** It's not marketing hype. Products designed to maintain the color in color-treated hair can help prevent fading, keep color true, and put back needed hydration.

- **Invest in a water filter you can attach to your showerhead.** It'll remove from the water minerals like chlorine, which can fade or distort your color (turning it green or brassy). You can get basic ones for less than $20 and more advanced versions for up to $120.

So now you know...

what a good investment hair color can be, how to make a good investment, and how to get the best returns on your hair color investment. So let's revisit hair color that makes you look like you don't have a dime and hair color that makes you look like a million bucks!

HAIR COLOR THAT MAKES YOU LOOK LIKE

You Don't Have a Dime

- Streaky, striped highlights

- Highlights without lowlights (the giant highlight syndrome)

- Solid, shoe-polish hair color

- Over-the-top, look-at-me hair color

- Hair color so perfect it looks fake

- Platinum, overbleached blonde

- Hair color too far from your natural hue, with obvious roots to prove it

- Red hair that's dull and faded

- Ashy, mousy brown hair that doesn't enhance your skin tone

- Color that clashes with your skin tone

HAIR COLOR THAT MAKES YOU LOOK LIKE

A Million Bucks

- Buttery or baby blonde-on-blonde highlights that are well-maintained

- Multidimensional hair with highlights and lowlights

- Highlights so fine and blended you can hardly see them (understated chic)

- Sun-kissed highlights that look like they came from nature

- Color with a glossy, shimmery finish

- Ombré highlights that start at the ends and work their way up

- Color that's grounded and natural-looking with depth (your own base color) at the nape, root, and on the underneath layers

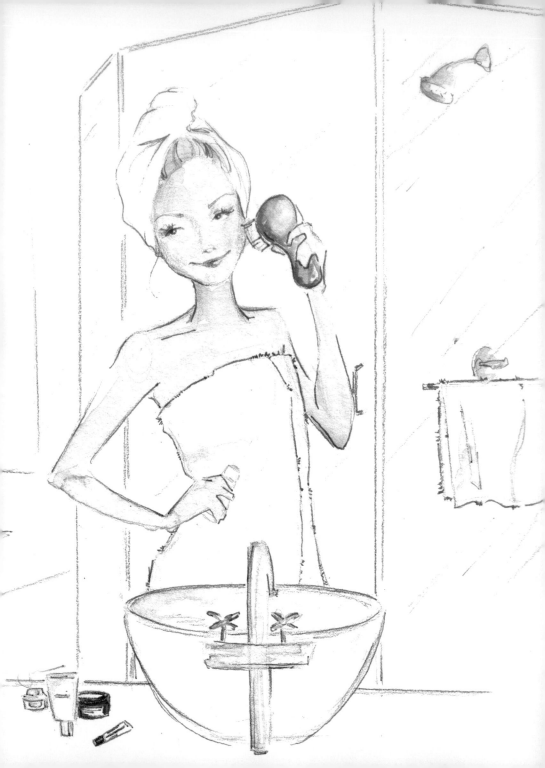

3

Beautiful
*Bare*able Skin

—— *The Ultimate Extravagance You Can Afford* ——

There are few greater luxuries than having beautiful, glowing skin. Skin so clear and luminous you want to show it off instead of slather it with makeup. Skin you want to get out and flaunt instead of fear in the mirror, and there are many reasons why. Great skin is right up there with killer arms and toned triceps as something to boast about. The most important? It's the ultimate expression of good health. And isn't health the ultimate kind of wealth? Another reason is that good skin used to be a little out of reach, unless you were twenty, genetically blessed, and lived the lifestyle of a saint (no smoking, no drinking, lots of sleep, a healthy diet, and never going to bed in your makeup), but that was before there was a revolution in the skin care industry—the end of the "hope in a jar" era and the beginning of skin care based on scientifically proven topical ingredients that really work.

The latest skin care products and procedures actually can change the structure of skin, put pimples out of business, and prevent and reverse aging. That's why many women see their skin doc more often than their dentist or even their hairstylist! Skin care advances have made 30 the new 20, 40 the new 30, and 50 the new 40, and turned all those beautiful celebrity faces that never seem to age (Hello, Sandra Bullock, Elle Macpherson, and countless other famous and non-famous forty-plus women who look half their age, we're talking about you!) into living, breathing billboards for flawless, ageless skin.

Now if you're thinking you have to be part of the 1 percent to have healthy, glowing skin, you're wrong. Healthy, glowing skin is achievable no matter your budget. It's not about the triple digits you spent on your antiaging product—great products can be found at all price points, if you know what to buy—the hoity-toityness of your dermatologist, or the fancy facial you can afford to splurge on, but rather that you get to know and take care of your skin. As Los Angeles facialist Stacy Cox says, "If you water the flowers, they grow; it's the same with skin. If you put in the effort, you'll reap the rewards." Let's review the difference between skin that looks expensive and skin that just *costs* a lot.

> *Skin care advances have made 30 the new 20, 40 the new 30, and 50 the new 40.*

Expensive-Looking Skin Versus Expensively Priced Skin

The Expensive Skin You Want!

This is skin that looks expensive but doesn't look like you spent a lot of money on treatments or tried too hard to get it. Instead, it looks like your skin just *is* healthy, fresh, glowing, and radiant. This kind of expensive skin is clear (no breakouts), dewy (a skin care word for moist), smooth (in texture), and even (in tone). It looks well-cared for, but in an understated, natural, self-loving way, not a high-maintenance or over-Botoxed, desperate housewife kind of way. Which brings me to . . .

The Expensive Skin You Don't Want!

This is skin that looks expensive because it actually *did* cost a fortune. It's skin that inadvertently advertises what's been done to it: the high-priced treatments like chemical peel after chemical peel that leave your skin as red and flaky as a red onion; fillers that transform your cheeks into tennis balls or make your lips look like inflated balloons; or Botox that leaves your face looking as though you live in Antarctica. It's skin that looks "bought," the opposite of natural, the face of a woman who needs a good therapist more than she needs another jar of La Mer or a shot of Restylane. This is *not* the kind of expensive skin advice you'll find here because it is the *opposite* of the less is more, understated elegance approach that is the goal of this book.

What Kind of Skin Makes You Look Cheap?

- Skin that hasn't been well-cared for, and the resulting sun damage, breakouts, blackheads, bumps, premature wrinkles, sallowness, and uneven tone and texture are the visible proof of the lack of attention.

- Skin that's shiny (as in oily) instead of dewy. You may not be able to help if your skin is naturally oily, but there are products out there designed to balance it.

- Skin that makes you look older than you are, maybe because it's a road map of negative lifestyle choices that all show up on your skin (it is, after all, your body's largest organ), like an unhealthy diet, drinking too much, smoking, drugs, and not enough sleep.

If you're having flashbacks to the last time you looked at your skin in the mirror, don't get mad, get even (skin, that is). Seriously. The good news about problem skin is it's a great starting point for changes. I recommend you take a picture of your skin right now before you begin to improve it, then take follow-up pictures every two weeks. And if you pull out that high-pixel digital camera to do it, all the better!

Gorgeous Skin Glossary

Understanding the Basics

I don't speak fluent French or Spanish but I do speak *Skin,* which I admit can sometimes seem like a foreign language! No worries—these confusing terms and products will be flowing off your tongue in no time. Until then, I'll use a familiar wardrobe analogy to make things easier for you.

There are so many skin care options out there, but you don't need all of them any more than you need a closet full of designer duds. The trick is to clear out the clutter and spend your money on the bare necessities that really work—then add on as your skin's needs determine or budget allows.

THE DAILY ESSENTIALS

These are your must-haves, equivalent in your wardrobe to the perfect white T-shirt, skinny jeans, cardigan sweater, LBD, and black leggings. You need to have all of these items in your wardrobe but if you choose the right version, you won't need more than one of each. This should be your goal with daily essentials—finding the right fit in terms of your skin's needs, the price point you are most comfortable with, and the look and feel that works for you.

CLEANSERS—Cleansing your face doesn't mean sudsing up with a bar of soap, which can actually strip your skin and make even oily skin feel dry. Better options are face cleansers without the drying surfactant (soap) ingredient, sodium lauryl sulfate. I especially like chemical-free cleansers that use natural, plant-based ingredients to do the dirty work. You don't need to overspend on cleanser—you wash it right off, so why bother? I like to shop at Whole Body or in the natural aisle of the drugstore for well-priced cleansers from brands like Alba Botanica, Avalon Organics, MyChelle Dermaceuticals, and Burt's Bees.

EXFOLIATORS—Also called scrubs, exfoliators are an important part of your regime. They can be used daily if your skin is normal to oily; two or three times a week if your skin is dry. They slough off grime and dead cells, either by physically removing them with grainy particles, buffing them away, or dissolving them invisibly with a mild acid (alpha hydroxy acid) or enzymatic scrub or wipe. I prefer the dissolving method. Exfoliators not only give you a fresh glow, but they also help products you put on afterward absorb better and work more efficiently.

MOISTURIZERS—
Dermatologist Ellen Marmur of New York's Mount Sinai Hospital tells me, "A good moisturizer is still right up there with sunscreen as one of the best antiaging products on the planet! It acts as a layer of protection that stops your body's own moisture from evaporating, allowing your skin to replenish from within naturally." Moisturizers sometimes include sunscreen, but if they don't, you need to apply sunscreen separately.

SUNSCREEN—Your coat of armor. Your workhorse. The number one antiager.

I know it's boring and hopefully I'm preaching to the converted, but I can't say enough about the importance of sunscreen for protecting your precious visage from the soleil! Some facial sunscreens are included in moisturizers, while others come in thin, liquidy formulas that slide on and disappear into your skin without interfering with your makeup or making you smell like cocoa butter at the office. I also like the new powder sunscreens with a built-in brush you just swipe on like face powder. (Perfect to store in a convertible for on-the-go protection!) The key attributes to look for in *any* sunscreen? Broad spectrum and SPF 30 or higher. And if you tend to break out from sunscreen, stick to hypoallergenic sunscreens that block rays physically instead of chemically via the ingredients titanium dioxide or zinc oxide in a micronized clear form.

EYE CREAM—Your under-eye skin is the thinnest on your body and

that's why it tends to show fine lines first. It's also why you get dark circles—the skin's thin veins play peekaboo. Dermatologists recommend eye creams to help plump up skin so you can't see the veins and to protect the area from losing moisture, a prime cause of crow's-feet. Dr. Ellen Marmur tells me the eye cream you choose doesn't matter and suggests going to the drugstore for this product, because the main goal is to prevent natural moisture from evaporating and any eye cream on the market will do that.

THE SKIN CARE SPANX: TREATMENT AND ANTIAGING PRODUCTS

These are the undercover secret weapons, the skin-controlling "lingerie and underpinnings" that will help you build and keep your skin looking luxe and healthy. Often referred to as "cosmeceuticals," treatment and antiaging products contain one or more active ingredients that can really change your skin. Cosmeceuticals come in different forms (serums, lotions, creams) and sometimes also contain moisturizing ingredients and/or sunscreens (buying one with all three can be a great way to economize). Use after cleansing, before sunscreen, unless your treatment product/antiager contains sunscreen, in which case you don't need a separate step. Some companies offer two treatment products with different active ingredients meant to be used in unison, either both at once as a lightweight serum you can layer under a heavier lotion or cream, or separately—the lighter one in the morning and the heavier one at night. Here's a look at some of the key active ingredients you'll find in these products. Pay attention to what they do, because you'll notice they have different functions on different skin types and can improve a multitude of skin concerns, be it acne or aging.

RETINOLS—The prescription-strength version of retinol, Retin-A, is the only FDA-approved antiaging ingredient proven to diminish fine lines and signs of aging, as well as clear up and improve acne. Less-concentrated versions of the ingredient can be found in skin care products at all price points. Every skin doc I've ever met wants you to incorporate Retin-A or one of its over-the-counter cousins into your routine (always at night because it can cause irritation).

What retinols can do for breakout-prone skin:
By exfoliating away dead cells and sebum (the natural oily substance found on our skin, which in excess can cause acne), retinols can help unclog pores and stimulate growth of collagen and elastin, your skin's internal support structure. Fewer breakouts, less acne scarring, and smaller pore size are the result.

What retinols can do for dry or aging skin: That same exfoliating action sloughs and mildly irritates skin, which sands away wrinkles so they look less deep. This irritation causes the skin to produce new collagen to repair itself, making new skin look younger and fresher. (The irritant effect can also cause redness and flaking. That's why when using a strong retinol-like prescription-strength Retin A, dermatologists recommend applying it at night and only every other night.)

LABEL SHOPPER
—
Retinol ingredients you'll find in over-the-counter skin care products include retinoic acid (the prescription Retin-A), retinaldehyde, retinoid, L-retinol AGP, retinol, vitamin A.

Retinol cautions: Avoid palmitate, a retinol ingredient recently found to be a possible carcinogen, and if you're pregnant or thinking of becoming pregnant, avoid all retinols until speaking with your doctor—certain ones have been found to possibly interfere with fetal development.

ALPHA HYDROXY ACIDS AND BETA HYDROXY ACIDS—These are mild acids derived from natural sources like milk, honey, citrus fruits, and apples. The major difference between AHAs and BHAs is their solubility. BHAs are oil-soluble, which means they're able to penetrate oil-clogged pores and clear them out. AHAs are water-soluble so they won't penetrate the pore directly but instead work on the surface to gently and invisibly slough away dead cells exposing a fresher layer of skin.

What AHAs/BHAs can do for breakout-prone skin: These mild acids gently exfoliate dead cells, getting into the cells to clean them out, which helps clear acne and blackheads. Salicylic acid is the most used BHA and is one of the most effective antiacne ingredients out there.

What AHAs/BHAs can do for normal to dry or aging skin: AHAs work as exfoliants to unglue and remove the dead cells on your skin's surface. This leaves behind a fresh layer of skin and may even help stimulate collagen and elastin production, two key ingredients of younger skin.

LABEL SHOPPER
—
AHA and BHA ingredients you'll find in skin care products include lactic acid, glycolic acid, malic acid, and salicylic acid.

ANTIOXIDANTS—These are ingredients that help neutralize the damage to your skin cells from environmental causes such as pollution, smoking, sun exposure, and alcohol, and in doing so hopefully help stall skin aging. Some skin care experts say they're as important as sunscreen and may even have a sunscreening effect, which is why they are popping up in both daily use and sunscreen products.

What antioxidants do for breakout-prone skin: By counteracting inflammation in your skin caused by environmental effects, antioxidants help prevent

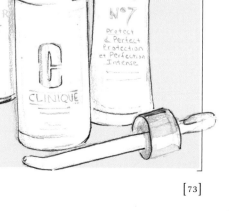

acne and calm and heal breakouts, while protecting your skin from premature aging.

What antioxidants do for normal to dry or aging skin: Antioxidants can help skin maintain moisture as well as combat the environmental assaults that cause skin to age (smoking, sun and pollution exposure).

PEPTIDES—Peptides are amino-acid chains that occur naturally in your skin and help build collagen and healthy skin. They're often added to skin care products in the hopes that they'll do the same thing when applied topically.

What peptides do for breakout-prone skin: Adding topical peptides may help reduce redness and prevent and improve the appearance of acne scars by aiding skin in the collagen-building process.

What peptides do for normal to dry or aging skin: Peptides, the building blocks of skin itself, may help repair aged skin so it looks thicker (like young skin) and less creased, while stimulating collagen production. Some products with peptides claim to have a line-relaxing function, kind of like topical Botox. Check reviews before you buy one of these, and don't expect miracles as there's some controversy on whether they work.

THE SKIN CARE "ACCESSORIES"

Like accessories in your wardrobe, these are optional extras that can

make a big impact. But also like accessories, if you overdo it, you easily can go from chic to eek! In other words, pick and choose from this category. You'll find that some of these are optional daily "essentials," while others are more special-occasion products and treatments that can supercharge your skin care routine at home.

FACIALS—Formerly the domain of the facialist/esthetician, there are now two kinds of facials—the traditional pampering kind (steam, extract, mask) and the more medical kind (usually involving some kind of acid peel or a laser). Even the more medical ones are sometimes given by estheticians. If you get a medical facial outside a doctor's office, be sure your esthetician is well-trained and experienced. I've heard horror stories of strip-mall laser and peel treatments and, personally, for anything more than a light peel, I would go to a doctor's office or "medical spa." Which to choose, pampering or medical? I honestly think medical facials are more worth the splurge; they're not as relaxing because they take only ten to twenty minutes and there's not a lot of lovey-dovey massage, but the results are often super-charged and longer lasting, giving you that skin-confident feeling that's actually its own kind of stress relief!

MASKS—A good mask can make you feel like a million bucks but, honestly, you don't really need one. Think of masks—be they hydrating, oil-absorbing, or balancing—as an extra you can use to pamper your skin, to rescue it from the blahs, or to revitalize and prepare it for a big event.

PEELS—Like a super-powered exfoliator, peels are secret skin-savers that use mild to more intense alpha hydroxy or beta hydroxy acids (often naturally derived) to peel away the superficial, tired outer layer of your skin, leaving behind a fresh new radiant layer, while also stimulating your skin to moisturize itself from within. Before I tell you about the options, a friendly word of caution: Done right and at the frequency recommended on the package or by a skin care expert, a peel can give you the texture, tone, and glow of expensive skin. When abused, it can do just the opposite.

DIY peels usually involve pads you wipe on and wipe off a few times a week; these fall back into the "daily essential" category and take the place of your exfoliator. Some contain alpha hydroxy acid for a skin-radiance effect; others contain salicylic acid for a skin-purifying, antiacne effect.

Professional peels contain a higher acid concentration and are offered as medical facials by both estheticians and dermatologists (remember, I always prefer the doctor) and can leave your skin invisibly but dramatically fresher. (These are called peels but at this level, the "peeling" is still invisible.)

More intense chemical peels offered by dermatologists exclusively utilize either the same ingredients at much higher strengths or stronger acids. These more serious peels, used mostly on more mature skin, cause skin to visibly peel off after a few days, leaving you housebound until what looks like a third-degree sunburn heals into fresh-looking skin. Again, fine in moderation and when performed by an experienced professional.

MICRODERMABRASION—Microdermabrasion is a great way to get expensive-looking, radiant, glowing skin. These treatments are similar to peels except they work by way of a gentle physical buffing action instead of a chemical peeling reaction. The premise behind microdermabrasion is that by softly "sanding" the skin, you'll increase cell turnover, stimulating skin to replace itself and produce collagen. Results include a reduction in the discoloration and indentation of acne scars and premature aging signs, more even skin tone, and minimized fine lines. Like peeling, you can do it yourself in lieu of at-home exfoliation, or have a more intense version performed at a dermatologist's office or skin spa.

Some options at both levels:

Sonic skin-cleansing machines, like Clarisonic face brushes or the similar and more economical Neutrogena WAVE Sonic, offer lighter forms of microdermabrasion, almost like a vibrating buff puff, that can be used daily to deep-cleanse the skin, taking the place of both cleanser and exfoliator.

Microdermabrasion pads are manual buffers you use in gentle circular motions with your hands to slough the skin's surface no more than once a week if skin is dry, three times a week if the skin is oily. They also negate the need for a separate exfoliator. RoC Daily Resurfacing Disks fall into this category, as do the more exclusive Intensify Facial Discs from Colbert MD, which I use myself. (They're more expensive, but they replicate a trip to the dermatologist's office, making them worth the splurge for me.)

At-home microderm-abrasion kits like the less than $20 Neutrogena Microdermabrasion System can be used once a week (they're stronger than the brushes or pads), taking the place of an exfoliator.

Professional microderm-abrasion is the strongest and most expensive, but will yield better results, too. You shouldn't have this done more than once a year.

CORTISONE SHOTS— If you've got a big pimple and a big date, a dermatologist can inject it with cortisone, an anti-irritant that depuffs on contact. Instant relief can be pricey—expect to pay up to $100 for a single shot. But sometimes it's worth it if you have a big event, if only for the psychological benefits of not thinking about a pimple during your wedding or job interview.

For a less expensive anti-inflammatory fix, try over-the-counter hydrocortisone cream, or a few tablets of ibuprofen. This does the same thing, though it may take a few hours!

JUVÉDERM, RESTYLANE, RADIESSE, AND SCULPTRA AESTHETIC—

These are injectable dermal "fillers" made with ingredients like hyaluronic acid that occur naturally in your skin. Often referred to as "liquid face-lifts," they're used to restore or add back fullness lost with age to facial features, as well as to fill in lines, creases, and scars. They aren't permanent but last long enough that you want only a real pro with lots of experience and a refined aesthetic sense to inject you with them. It's important to note that a little filler can do wonders but too much can cost a bundle and it won't look expensive—it distorts your face until it wears off, a sight I've seen, and it's not very pretty.

LASER AND RADIO-FREQUENCY TREATMENTS—These

involve high-tech machines that your dermatologist may use to spot-treat various skin conditions, from broken capillaries to sun damage to rosacea to fine lines and wrinkles, even stretch marks and cellulite. Each device has a different effect, but most work via light or heat energy to zap problem spots and stimulate the skin to produce new collagen. Some require no downtime, and others offer more intense results but you have to hide out for a few days. Results become apparent over weeks or months. These high-tech "facials" can cost a lot ($250 to $1,500 per session) and need to be administered by a trained doctor, but they're a great option for women who are first starting to see aging signs and want to improve their skin without needles. For first-step antiaging treatments, ask your doctor about Clear + Brilliant, IPL facials, Thermage, and Gentle Waves. There are also laser and light treatments like Isolaz that dermatologists are really excited about because they improve acne.

BOTOX AND DYSPORT—

These are toxins that can be injected into your skin by a dermatologist to "freeze" frown lines between your brows, and wrinkles on your forehead and around your eyes. Results last for four months, but if not done correctly or overdone, you can permanently lose the ability to make certain facial movements, which new studies show can actually affect your emotions. (If you can't smile, you may not feel happy!) I like the idea of what Dr. Ellen Marmur calls "Baby Botox." Small amounts of it are applied in intervals across the forehead to rid horizontal forehead wrinkles without the can't-move-your-eyebrows side effect. That's the trick to getting toxins to look expensive: Use as little as possible.

Your Easiest, Most Effective Daily Skin Care Regime

Now that you can decipher labels and company claims and find products that fit your budget, lifestyle, and skin care needs, it's time to find yourself an effective skin care regime. The most important thing I want you to remember is that luxe-looking skin starts at home! The key is caring for your skin consistently with a twice-daily regime that you can stick to. Here's what I recommend as a daily routine. Use the label shopper lists in the Gorgeous Skin Glossary and see some of my favorites on pages 80–81 to help you choose the products you need.

If You Have Normal to Oily Skin

In the morning

Cleanse: Use a cleanser to remove dead cells and sweat from the night before. Choose one you'll use because you like the smell or the way it makes your skin feel, and leave it in the shower so you don't forget to use it.

Treat/Moisturize: Pick a does-it-all skin care serum or lotion that contains antioxidants and/or sunscreen. *Optional:* Eye cream (or just use the serum or lotion under—but not touching—your eyes).

Protect: If your serum or lotion doesn't contain sunscreen, add one on top. SPF 30 or higher, please, with broad-spectrum protection (should be clearly labeled as offering both).

In the evening

Cleanse: Use the same cleanser or use a makeup-removing wipe for haste and ease (sensitive-skin natural baby wipes are a good cheap option).

Wipe: I like to add an exfoliating "peel" pad (from the accessories list) to unclog pores, which gives my skin a fresh feel.

Treat: Use a serum or lotion product with salicyclic acid or retinols (even prescription Retin-A) to unblock pores. *Optional:* Add eye cream.

If You Have Normal to Dry or Aging Skin

In the morning

Cleanse: Skip cleanser in the morning and just freshen your face with water, a trick lots of female dermatologists use on themselves.

Treat: Use a serum, lotion, or cream that contains active ingredients like antioxidants, retinols, and peptides as well as moisturizing ingredients like hyaluronic acid or glycerine. Apply eye cream to your under-eye area, patting it in instead of rubbing.

Protect: Apply a sunscreen. If it has additional antioxidants or moisturizing ingredients, all the better, but what it must have is SPF 30 or higher and broad-spectrum protection (should be clearly labeled as offering both).

In the evening

Cleanse: Use a hydrating cleanser or skin-hydrating wipe to remove makeup, dead cells, and grime from the day.

Exfoliate: Once or twice a week use a gentle exfoliator, wipe, or pad that contains alpha hydroxy acid (AHA) to rid dead cells more thoroughly and expose fresher skin.

Treat: Use your morning serum, lotion, or cream, or use a night cream loaded with the same antiaging ingredients. Add prescription-strength Retin-A two or three times a week and use an eye cream every night.

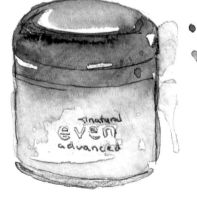

Shortcut to Great Skin

I'm personally more likely to follow a skin care routine if it's short and sweet. When I'm especially cash-strapped or busy, I'll minimize the routine above by picking multipurpose products that let you skip a step or even two or three, say, an AHA cleanser that exfoliates and cleanses, followed by a moisturizing treatment product with sunscreen that can also work as an eye cream when needed. Many of the products I recommend on the next page can help you multitask.

Andrea's Skin Care A-List

*These are some of my favorite products at all price levels, and I've given
you some natural choices, too. Note that I've included manufacturer list prices,
but many of these products can be found online for less.*

MY FAVORITE
Eye Creams/Gels

High-end: EltaMD Renew Eye Gel Daily Eye Therapy, $45–49

Natural: Burt's Bees Naturally Ageless Smoothing Eye Cream, $25

Drugstore: L'Oréal Paris Youth Code Eye Cream, $24.99; RoC Retinol Correxion Sensitive Eye Cream, $22.99

MY FAVORITE
Cleansers

High-end for Oily Skin: Dermalogica Dermal Clay Cleanser, $33

High-end for Normal to Dry Skin: Estée Lauder Perfectly Clean Splash Away Foaming Cleanser, $20

Natural for Oily Skin: Origins Zero Oil Deep Pore Cleanser with Saw Palmetto and Mint, $19.50

Natural for Normal to Dry Skin: Alba Botanica Even Advanced Sea Lettuce Cleansing Milk, $10.99; Alba Botanica Hawaiian Coconut Facial Wash, $12.95

Drugstore for Oily Skin: CeraVe Foaming Facial Cleanser, $12.99

Drugstore for Normal to Dry Skin: Neutrogena Naturals Fresh Cleansing + Makeup Remover, $7.49; Aveeno Ultra-Calming Foaming Cleanser, $6.99

MY FAVORITE
Facial Sunscreens for Daily Use

High-end: StriVectin-SH Age Protect SPF 30, $49; Neova DNA Damage Control Everyday SPF 43, $39; Colorescience PRO Sunforgettable Mineral Powder Sun Protection SPF 30 Brush, $50

Natural: MyChelle Dermaceuticals Sun Shield SPF 28, $19.19

Drugstore: Neutrogena Healthy Defense Liquid Moisturizer SPF 50, $12.99

MY FAVORITE
Moisturizers

High-end for Oily Skin: Bobbi Brown Oil Control Lotion SPF 15, $48

High-end for Normal to Dry Skin: Murad Sheer Lustre Day Moisture SPF 15, $68

Natural for Oily Skin: Aubrey Organics Natural Herbal Maintenance Oil Balancing Moisturizer, $14.15

Natural for Normal to Dry Skin: Alba Botanica Even Advanced Sea Moss Moisturizer SPF 15, $16.99

Drugstore for Oily Skin:
Garnier Nutritioniste Moisture Rescue Lightweight UV Lotion SPF 15, $5.99

Drugstore for Normal to Dry Skin: Aveeno Positively Radiant Daily Moisturizer SPF 30, $16

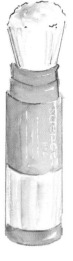

MY FAVORITE
Antiaging Products

High-end: Colbert MD Nutrify & Protect, $95, and Stimulate: The Serum, $135; 37 Extreme Actives by Dr. Alexiades, $295

Natural: Avalon Organics Essential Lift Lifting Serum, $25.95; Alba Botanica Even Advanced Sea Lipids Daily Cream, $16.99

Drugstore: RoC Multi Correxion Skin Renewing Serum, $24.99

MY FAVORITE
Peel Pads

High-end: Kate Somerville Clinic-to-Go Resurfacing Peel Pads, $48; Colbert MD Intensify Facial Discs, $52

Natural: Origins Brighter By Nature High-Potency Brightening Peel with Fruit Acids, $37.50; First Aid Beauty Facial Radiance Pads, $28

Drugstore: RoC Retinol Correxion Daily Resurfacing Disks, $9.99

MY FAVORITE
Pimple Fixers

High-end: GoClear Intensive Acne Treatment, $25

Natural: Yes to Tomatoes Clear Skin Spot Stick, $9.99

Drugstore: Clean & Clear Advantage Acne Spot Treatment, $6.49

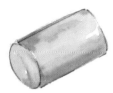

MY FAVORITE
Exfoliators

High-end: Kate Somerville ExfoliKate Intensive Exfoliating Treatment, $85; Tracie Martyn Enzyme Exfoliant, $90; Estée Lauder Idealist Dual-Action Refinishing Treatment, $49.50

Natural: Suki Exfoliate Foaming Cleanser, $29.95; Neutrogena Naturals Purifying Pore Scrub, $7.49

Drugstore: Olay Professional Pro-X Exfoliating Renewal Cleanser, $18.99

Four Skin Superheroes the Stars Swear By

BOOK AN APPOINTMENT WITH...

DR. DAVID COLBERT

The Celebrity Skin Doc Who Believes Beauty Is More Than Skin Deep

You'll find David Colbert in his loft-like office in New York City's busy Flatiron District. David's signature skin care line, Colbert MD, really works. But the best piece of advice David ever gave me had nothing to do with buying high-end products. He realized the reason his celeb clients like Michelle Williams and Sienna Miller looked so great was more than skin-deep: They were all eating low-glycemic, farm-fresh, locally sourced food whenever possible. I tried David's diet and not only did my skin start to glow but I also lost the ten pounds I'd gained while nursing a sprained ankle, as well as the dark circles under my eyes. This way of eating has transformed my life, my body, and my skin. Thanks, David!

David says his healthy-skin diet is better for your skin than Botox! That was all I had to hear to try it.

David's Pet Peeves

Tanning. "It makes me crazy because it reverses all the hard work we do to make the skin look and feel younger," he says.

Forgetting the neck, chest, arms, and hands, and only treating the face with skin care products. We want all those areas to look the same age, so he recommends using facial products on primo-visible body parts like hands, neck, and décolletage. This may sound expensive, but he thinks it's easier to prevent damage now than have to fix it later; buy a drugstore product for your body if you use an expensive one on your face.

David's Cheap Trick

Greek yogurt for breakfast. Dr. Colbert told me to do it, I did, and it works. Maybe all those probiotics calm your digestive system, which calms your skin from the inside out?

BOOK AN APPOINTMENT WITH...

NERIDA JOY

The Beverly Hills Facialist

Aussie Nerida Joy is an in-the-know secret in Beverly Hills, where she's honed her trade as an esthetician for more than two decades. Known for her calming, sensible advice, stars who swear by her include Jennifer Garner (who actually refers to Nerida as "magic"), Reese Witherspoon, Kate Beckinsale, and Courteney Cox, women with some of the best skin in the business. Nerida's facial technique is heavy on the massage, which she believes helps ingredients to penetrate. And in terms of what you should use at home, no matter your skin type or problem, oily, breakout prone, or aging and wrinkle prone, she says only four ingredients matter—retinols, alpha hydroxy acids, antioxidants, and peptides—the same four I told you about in the Skin Care Spanx section. For us mere mortals, she now consults online at BeautyMint.com

Even the stars can't take Nerida's hands home, so she recommends that you try massaging skin care products in yourself—the heat of your hands aids in penetration.

Nerida's Pet Peeve

Cosmetic procedure junkies. She believes cosmetic surgery/dermatology is actually addictive and women get hooked on even small procedures, thinking more is more rather than less is best. She gifts women who seem caught in the cycle with free copies of self-help, self-love CDs and books by Louise Hay and Dr. Wayne Dyer.

Nerida's Cheap Trick

Ice to shrink a pimple. She'd rather her stars use ice than get a cortisone shot at the dermatologist, which she finds helps in the short term but sometime leaves a pit when the skin heals.

BOOK AN APPOINTMENT WITH...

DR. BOBBY BUKA

The Skin Star Who Treats the Stars' Skin

Dr. Bobby Buka is a regular on the sets of New York–based television productions and loves the challenge of treating celebrities, often in tiny spaces with terrible lighting and just his little black bag. Buka is another big believer in topical treatments with supercharged antioxidants (his favorite is licorice root) to counteract collagen breakdown. He says it's never too early to start to use them and he actually has his own line of well-priced, down-to-earth, and healthy-for-you (e.g., no parabens) skin products, called First Aid Beauty, sold at Sephora and frequently recommended by other dermatologists. When it comes to wrinkles, it's his subtle touch that keeps celebs flocking to his nest. And Dr. Buka's not one to overdo it with the fillers or toxins.

"I'll intentionally under-treat a patient using Botox by 5 to 10 percent less, so she doesn't look frozen, with the caveat that if she wants to come back for more, I won't charge more."

—Dr. Buka

WHY IT'S CHEAPER FOR YOU TO SEE DR. BUKA THAN IT IS FOR JENNIFER ANISTON

Next time you practically faint over a dermatologist or doctor's bill, consider this: Though a dermatologist will charge the same rate to you and celebrities like Jen, you don't have the added expense of asking him to clear out the waiting room a half hour before and after your appointment so you can slip through the back door unnoticed. "I have to calculate the mean income for that number of patients lost and then that cost gets passed on to the patient." Sounds fair, if insane, but Dr. Buka has no guilt: "They have the ability to pay more, so they do, with the studio usually picking up the bill."

Dr. Buka's Pet Peeve

Dermatologists who listen to their patients instead of themselves. "You pay for an expert, let him tell you what's right for you. And don't push your doctor to go further than he wants to. Less is always more," he says.

Dr. Buka's Cheap Tricks

Afrin nasal spray, as an antiredness treatment for irritated skin. "It's a vassal constrictor that will take the red out in less than an hour."

Ibuprofen after sun exposure to counteract the damage-causing free radicals released in your skin three hours after a burn.

A soft washcloth used in circular motions to mimic the deep-cleansing effect of a Clarisonic facial cleansing machine.

BOOK AN APPOINTMENT WITH...

STACY COX

The Down-to-Earth Skin Care Diva

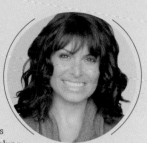

Stacy Cox's definition of an expensive complexion is skin that's bright, even-toned, supple, yet firm and looks younger than the age of the woman wearing it. Getting such skin, she believes, is all about self-love and desire, not the size of your wallet. It's about making the effort to have what she calls a BAP (beauty action plan) and sticking to it for decades. Stacy believes in mixing and matching drugstore and prestige like you would a T-shirt from Zara with a Michael Kors skirt you bought as an investment. She suggests skimping on cleanser, which stays on your skin for only minutes, and making a deeper financial investment in treatment and antiaging products with clinically proven pharmaceutical results. And I like Stacy's thirty-day rule: Used it for a month with no visible changes? Move on, it's a relationship going nowhere!

"Your wrinkles have taken your whole life to form, so give a new product more than a week to show results!"

—Stacy Cox

Stacy's Pet Peeve

"Women who have a bathroom counter littered with antiaging potions and only one face to use them on." If you don't want buyer's remorse, she suggests never going skin care shopping when you're having a down day or PMS, you're too vulnerable.

Stacy's Favorite Cheap Trick

A DIY kitchen-chemical peel to mimic the results you'd get from a dermatologist: Mix 3 tablespoons apple juice (malic acid, a gentle exfoliator), 3 tablespoons milk (lactic acid, a more intense exfoliator found in many antiaging products), and 1 egg white (to firm the skin). Apply for 15 to 20 minutes, then rinse with warm water.

A Celebrity Facial to Try at Home by Ole Henriksen

Ole Henriksen is an LA skin genius who hangs his hat on Hollywood Boulevard, not far from the famous Hollywood sign. What I like about Ole's treatments is that he uses all natural ingredients. I asked Ole for a home version of the facial he gives stars like Cameron Diaz and Jessica Alba before the Oscars to make their skin shine as bright as their star power. Take it away, Ole!

OLE'S CELEBRITY FACIAL SHOPPING LIST

Buy these natural ingredients at Whole Foods or on Amazon.com to make Ole's DIY recipes, or use your own mask and scrub, following his application instructions.

INGREDIENTS

- **Golden flaxseed powder** is plentiful in omega-3 essential fatty acids, which helps to add luminosity to the skin's texture while having gentle exfoliating benefits.

- **Himalayan pink salt** is a great deep-cleansing exfoliant, providing the skin with important minerals.

- **Argan oil** provides for a smooth glide across the skin while also providing nourishment and conditioning via the perfect balance of essential fatty acids.

- **1 roll of gauze**

- **1 cucumber**

- **Aromatherapeutic candles**

- **1 box rooibos tea** (African red tea)

- **1 jar lavender-infused honey**

"When creating an at-home spa experience, it is very important to set the mood in your bathroom and have everything ready ahead of time, including any homemade skin recipes. This will allow you to flow from treatment step to treatment step in a relaxed manner, putting all your focus and energy into your personal pampering."

—Ole Henriksen

THE FACIAL

1. LIGHT AROMA-THERAPY CANDLES, put on soft music, and gather all the ingredients for your treatments, as well as a terry facecloth, towel, and a rolled hand towel for under the neck.

2. FILL YOUR SINK a third of the way with lukewarm water. Brew 2 cups (16 ounces) of rooibos tea using 2 tea bags and add this to the water in the sink. This basically becomes like a facial steam, enhancing circulation and providing the skin with rich antioxidants. Drench your terry facecloth in this aromatic mixture and press against the face, holding it in place for 30 seconds at a time, relaxing your upper body, repeating a total of 5 to 10 times.

3. APPLY OLE'S PINK HIMALAYAN COMPLEXION SCRUB (made ahead of time), working the mixture into the skin in gentle outward, upward circular motions, making sure to get into every corner of the face to polish, refine, and deep cleanse all in one.

4. MASSAGE 2 tablespoons of the lavender-infused honey (honey is full of natural antioxidants, moisturizers, and is antibacterial, making it the perfect mask for all skin types), and massage it into the face in upward, outward motions. Then lay down on your towel with an additional towel rolled beneath your neck to support your head. Place the cucumber rolls over your eyes and lay with your legs slightly parted and arms gently at your sides, palms facing up for about ten minutes. Relax, breathe, enjoy.

5. RINSE THE HONEY OFF with a warm washcloth to gently but thoroughly melt it off your skin. Then stare at your glow in the mirror!

OLE'S PINK HIMALAYAN COMPLEXION SCRUB

1. Mix 1 tablespoon of golden flaxseed powder, 1 tablespoon of Himalayan pink salt, 1½ tablespoons of argan oil.

2. Stir the ingredients together and store in an airtight Tupperware container in the fridge. When ready to use, pour a little less than 2 teaspoons into a small bowl, stir to refresh, and bring it into the bathroom.

RELAXING CUCUMBER DEPUFFING EYE GAUZE

Grate a cucumber and dividing the flesh and juice evenly, roll it up into two separate strips of gauze to create a mask for each eye. This optimizes the cucumber juice, allowing it to seep through for the greatest depuffing action.

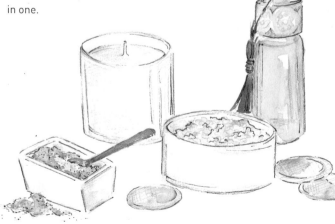

The New Red-Carpet Secret Weapon

Single-use masks you apply to your skin for ten minutes (while you rest or do your hair) for serious hydrating results. Celebs use these while sitting in their makeup trailers, apartments, and hotel rooms, glamming up for parties and close-ups. The idea was originally imported from Japan, and the masks are usually made of some kind of stretchy paper drenched in active ingredients such as collagen itself, glow-inducing gems or electromagnetically charged gold particles (increases blood flow for a glow), antioxidant red-wine extract, vitamin C, or superpower moisturizer hyaluronic acid. Some of these single-use masks cover your whole face, others just your eye area, and though a mask you can only use once may not seem economical at first, when you consider that they give you the results of a pre-party professional facial ($60 to $250, depending on where you live), $5 to $20 each becomes almost cheap. But the results they give? Expensive!

SPLURGE

Koh Gen Do Macro Vintage Essence Mask, 6 for $110; Wei Gingko Leaf Repairing Face Treatment Pads, 6 for $68; Christine Valmy Gold Collagen Mask, $16.50 each; Bliss Triple Oxygen Instant Energizing Eye Masks, 4 for $54

SAVE

Caswell-Massey Revitalizing Cool Cucumber Eye Pads, 24 for $12; DuWop igels, 3 pairs for $25; Kose Clear Turn White Marine Collagen Paper Facial Mask, 5 for $13.98 on Amazon.com; Mayblesally Vitamin C System L-ascorbic Acid Whitening Hydrating Cloth Mask, $5.75 each on Amazon.com

SKIN CARE FREEBIES FROM THE WORLD'S MOST EXPENSIVE FACIALIST

Celebrities like Kate Winslet swear by British-born facialist Tracie Martyn to keep their skin glowing—without any invasive needles or procedures. An hour on her table can take ten years off your skin: You look glowing and gorgeous—like you had a face-lift. That's why, at $550 a session, her followers call it a bargain. But reaping the benefits of her advice doesn't require a black Amex. Here are some free Tracie tips to try.

• **Drink plenty of water,** but between meals, not during them, to avoid diluting digestive enzymes that pull toxins from your skin.

• **Stay away from refined sugar.** The sweet stuff binds to collagen and destroys it. And before celeb clients walk the red carpet, she tells them to avoid excess sodium and alcohol, which can cause water retention and puffiness.

• **Eat lots of antioxidants.** Red, blue, and purple foods protect the skin.

• **Relax.** Biochemically, when you reach an alpha state of relaxation during sleep or meditation (Tracie gets her clients there on her table), it's proven to make a big difference in your skin. "You produce different endorphins and peptides when you relax that repair and regenerate collagen and elastin," she says.

• **Defy gravity by sleeping on your back, not your face.** Tracie herself sleeps with two pillows on each side of her head. "It makes a difference year after year when you wake up with a face that's not all smushed."

CREATIVE WAYS TO GET MORE BANG
FOR YOUR SKIN CARE BUCKS

Buy skin care products online. Besides offering discounted products, you can also access reviews and advice. Sites like LovelySkin.com, run by a famous dermatologist, offer great money-saving options, oversize samples, and advice from trained skin experts online and over the phone. On Sephora.com and even Amazon.com, you can read skin care reviews before you hit the checkout box.

Shop Costco for high-end skin care products at discount prices. The same bulk buying strategy that gets you toilet paper for less works for skin products, too.

Pay up to pay less. Spring for the expensive in-office procedure instead of cycling through multiple products that aren't as effective. You'll get more bang for your buck in terms of results, plus you won't be tempted to buy every new product to fix a problem that will no longer exist.

Save on cleansers and skip toners. See my recommended drugstore cleansers and skip the toners, which most skin pros say are useless anyway. I like to use inexpensive baby wipes for sensitive skin to give me the clean-skin feel of a toner.

Mix it up. Like fashion, where you may shop at a discount or department store, you can go high-end, low-end, and everywhere in between with your skin care products—and wear them all at the same time. A cleanser from Whole Body, a treatment product from Proactiv, with a sunscreen from Clarins? Why not! Though companies will try to get you to buy the whole regime, doing so can be as boring as walking into Chanel and saying, "I'll take the whole head-to-toe look, shoes and all."

Streamline the products in your skin care regime. With more products combining active ingredients, it's easy to get all your skin needs in two or three products. Plus, I find the less I use, the more likely I am to stick with it.

Don't be a label whore. I'm referring to women who use the "it" expensive skin care product even if it doesn't work for them, kind of like buying a pair of "it" jeans that make you look fat . . . not worth the splurge!

Get a prescription acne or rosacea medication. It's bound to be more effective than its drugstore counterpart, and it may even cost less because insurance might pay for it! Ask your dermatologist about Differin, Acanya, Tazorac, azelaic acid, and clindamycin.

Princess-Perfect Skin on a Pauper's Budget

Notice how Kate Middleton never has bags under her eyes, dark circles, blackheads, or a greasy T-zone? How her skin is always the perfect peaches-and-cream complexion, always even and glowing, never red, dry, or dull? Here's how to quickly fix a myriad of skin problems to get skin as rich as royalty without breaking the bank (or marrying a prince).

PROBLEM

Shine that's more greasy than gorgeous

FIX

Blot with a Starbucks napkin. Something about their weave and texture makes them the perfect face-blotters!

PROBLEM

Large visible pores

FIXES

Use pore-minimizing foundation or primer, like Clinique Pore Refining Solutions Instant Perfector, $18; Dr. Brandt Pores No More Pore Refiner Hint of Tint, $45; or Rimmel London Fix & Perfect Foundation Primer, $8.99.

PROBLEM

Blackheads

FIXES

Bioré Deep Cleansing Pore Strips, $7.99. Still the best. Or make your own with this recipe from YouTube star Michelle Phan, which I've included in my *Glamour* column: Mix 1 tablespoon each of unflavored gelatin and milk; microwave for 10 seconds. Let cool and apply to your nose. When the gelatin is dry and has hardened against your skin, peel off in a strip.

PROBLEM

Skin looks dull, tired

FIXES

Get moving! Twenty minutes of aerobic exercise will rev up circulation and bring color and life to your skin. Or do just the opposite: sleep! One skin doc says seven to nine hours at least four nights a week is equivalent to getting filler injections and the Fraxel laser . . . and maybe even a little Botox!

PROBLEM

Redness or irritation

FIX

Afrin nasal spray. Dr. Bobby Buka suggests applying a few drops to your fingertips and rubbing it over reddened skin.

PROBLEM

Zits

FIXES

Take ibuprofen to reduce swelling internally and hydrocortisone cream to reduce swelling topically. Or crush a few aspirin to form a powder, add water to make a paste, apply to zits before bed, then cover with Band-Aids.

PROBLEM

Dry, flaky patches

FIXES

Apply a little lip balm, rubbed in with your fingertips. Or a thin layer of Vaseline or olive oil will do the trick, too.

PROBLEM

Dark circles

FIXES

Dr. Bobby Buka recommends his celeb clients soak gauze in soy milk and apply it as a mask an hour before bed. Another idea: Make ice cubes out of green tea and defrost two cubes by massaging them one at a time beneath each eye.

PROBLEM

Under-eye bags

FIXES

You can take an antihistamine like Allegra to reduce swelling (which is often a sign of irritation). Also helpful: Freeze two squares of Jell-O in plastic wrap and use them as compresses, or apply two steeped and chilled black tea bags to your eyes. And I know this sounds weird, but Dr. Ellen Marmur, a very serious dermatologist, recommends it: After a night of sushi or french fries, when you know you'll be puffy in the morning, put some first-aid paper tape under your eyes. It'll keep the water away from your eyes so you wake up without any baggage from the night before!

Cult Celebrity Skin Care Secrets

Celebrities and their dermatologists have lots of tricks up their sleeves to make skin gorgeous. And yes, they can be super pricey. But they don't have to be. Take a look at these high-priced skin care secrets . . . and some money-saving ways to get the same effects for less.

SPLURGE

Dr. Sebagh Serum Repair, $140
-or-
Trish McEvoy Beauty Booster Serum, $125

These super-high-powered, skin-plumping formulas contain a high concentration of hyaluronic acid, which is the high-charged moisturizing ingredient your skin makes naturally and the basis for fillers like Restylane. Use it like a moisturizer before a special date or event.

SAVE

You can buy pure hyaluronic acid on Amazon.com for about $20.

SPLURGE

The Clarisonic Opal, $185

Before a television appearance, stars use this sonic-infusion machine to temporarily fill wrinkles. You place the device under your eye, push a button, and it pulsates for twenty seconds, infusing a special marine-derived antiaging formula into your skin.

SAVE

Preparation H!

It's also used by celebrities as an instant wrinkle fix. You just apply a little under your makeuplike eye cream or moisturizer. The catch is you need to buy the Canadian version (easily done on Amazon.com) because the United States took out the ingredient with the antiwrinkle effect (live yeast extract) because it didn't seem to help hemorrhoids! About $21.

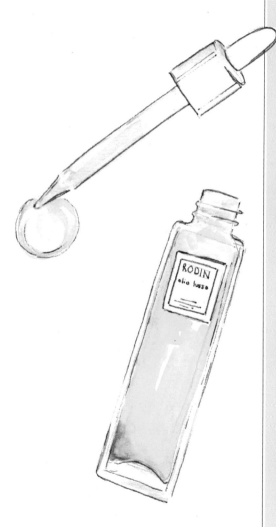

SPLURGE

RODIN Olio Lusso Luxury Face Oil, $140

I first heard about this high-end blend of eleven delicious-smelling oils, created by an ultra-chic, longtime globe-trotting fashion stylist, from top model Chanel Iman. A few drops are all you need to give skin a dewy glow—the $140 bottle goes a long way. For me, it doubles as perfume, making it worth the splurge. To apply, just dab it on your fingertips or into your palms, then massage it into your skin.

SAVE

Olive oil!

It too will give skin a dewy glow. Skin care guru Kate Somerville tells me she uses olive oil on her skin a few times a week, and my makeup artist friend Julie Morgan, who glams up chef Giada De Laurentiis, uses a pinch on Giada's skin for a fresh radiance in and out of the kitchen. If you're not into smelling like a salad, I also love Lierac Paris Huile Sensorielle Aux 3 Fleurs, a beautiful botanical multiuse oil sold at the drugstore for about $34.

SPLURGE

Tracie Martyn LotuSculpt
Quick Fix Eye Pad Activator, $50
-with-
Tracie Martyn LotuSculpt Re Sculpt
Quick Fix Eye Pads, $45

This peptide-rich formula smoothes, de-puffs, and brightens dark circles, and can be used with or without the eye pads, which turn it into a strip mask.

SAVE

Earth Therapeutics Hydrogel
Under-Eye Recovery Patch,
set of 5 for $7.99

SPLURGE

NARS the Multiple in Orgasm, $39

A cream peachy-gold blush stick to fake the glow when you just can't make it happen. I dab it onto the apples of my cheeks, then blend it in with my fingertips. Don't be surprised when you read about this again in the makeup chapter—it's my can't-live-without passion.

SAVE

Maybelline New York Dream Bouncy
Blush in Hot Tamale, $7.99
(Apply with fingers.)

SPLURGE

Josie Maran 100% Pure Argan Oil, $48

Celebs love this natural antioxidant oil from a Moroccan tree because it absorbs immediately into your skin, leaving the prettiest glow. Dab a few drops on your fingertips and lightly blend into skin using circular motions.

SAVE

Do an Amazon.com search for argan oil and you'll find lots of organic options in the $10 to $28 range.

SPLURGE

The Clarisonic Skin Brush,
$119–$225

The skin care brush every expert raves about. Though not cheap, using it to cleanse your face daily keeps your skin so clear and clean you need fewer facials or trips to the dermatologist. Your products will also work more efficiently without running into a wall of clogged pores, which is priceless, don't you think? There's even a special version that is used with a salicylic acid cleanser that's great for acne-prone skin.

SAVE

Neutrogena Sonic Wave, $13.99;
Olay Professional Pro-X Advanced
Cleansing System, $29.99

The Rest of You: Making Every Inch of Your Skin Look Expensive

It's not enough to just pay attention to the skin on your face. Hands and neck are the next two places that show age, followed by décolletage. To stave off aging, stars actually get body facials or have body laser treatments. They are also scrupulous about sunscreen and often use facial skin treatment and antiaging products on their hands and necks, too! That can be pricey and time-consuming, but at the very least, you can rub the excess antiaging lotion you put on your face into the backs of your hands. I noticed that I had been dabbing my cream on my left hand from the tube before slathering it on my face, causing the skin on one hand to be significantly softer and less lined than the other! Try the one-hand test and you'll see what I mean. You can also downgrade to a less expensive facial product to use on your neck, décolletage, and hands . . . or use an old product you still own but have moved on from.

> *You can rub the excess antiaging lotion you put on your face into the back of your hands.*

My Favorite Body-Skin Softening Trick: Coconut Milk!

A can costs about $5 and you can easily turn it into the most luxurious, deliciously scented moisturizer in less than twenty-four hours. Just open the can and let it solidify in the fridge. It'll turn into a solid butter you can use on skin to make yourself silky soft. Keep it in the fridge and you'll be able to get just as much moisturizer out of that one can as a tube of expensive body cream . . . but it's natural and smells *beyond!*

One Expensive Habit That Gives You Permission to Be a Cheapskate!

When it comes to injectable fillers and Botox, you have my permission to cheap out, by which I mean, say no. It's not that I have anything against these treatments, just that there's lots of potential to look really weird for months on end if the doctors make a mistake. A little of one of these treatments can go a long way if you find a doctor with skill and taste, and you go in with the expectation that less is more. Still, you may find that with the right skin care products, you don't even need them. I've seen women who become unrecognizable even to close friends over time. Here's why: The first time you get Botox it looks great. But skin care procedures can be addictive and you begin to think "I want more," and at the next appointment you ask your doctor to go even further. But now your doctor is working from a different starting point and eventually you begin to look like someone other than yourself!

There's lots of potential to look really weird for months on end if the doctors make a mistake.

If you are going to try any procedure, a few tips to get the most natural results:

- **Ask about noninvasive laser and heat therapies to start.** A few, like the IPL and Thermage, offer great results with little downtime. And Fraxel is supposed to be a miracle treatment (it refreshes, restores, and reinvigorates collagen) with just a few days off (a weekend spent at home) and no strange "Who are you?" side effects.

- **Bring in pictures of your younger self to show your doctor.** It may help to have these on hand for reference to restore natural contours and fullness accurately. Even photos of your mother and grandmothers can help predict future aging.

- **A good doctor knows which wrinkles to get rid of and which ones to keep.** Look at your face with your dermatologist and figure out which ones are the keepers, instead of taking the wrinkle Wite-Out approach, which never looks natural.

So let's review.

You've now got so many more tools at your disposal to help you make smart skin care choices at whatever price you're most comfortable with. You know that beautiful skin takes effort. You also know that beautiful skin is the ultimate luxury, and that once you have it, you'll feel liberated, able to wear makeup or skip it. You'll feel younger and fresher. You'll look glowing and gorgeous with minimal effort and have the good skin confidence to go with it, perhaps the greatest gift you can give yourself. It's priceless!

WORK YOUR
Skin Care Budget

IF YOU HAVE $500 TO SPEND ON SKIN CARE

See a dermatologist for advice and put your money toward a professional peel. While you're there, pick his brain for the products that are best for your skin at a price/shopping venue you can afford.

-OR-

Get yourself three new skin care products (cleanse, treat, protect, or an eye cream or glycolic acid pads) and use what's left for a facial.

IF YOU HAVE $250 TO SPEND

Buy an at-home facial device designed to give professional results, such as a Clarisonic brush (it's genius, and a dermatologist-recommended must-have).

-OR-

Splurge on a professional facial—don't just fall asleep; interrogate the facialist for skin care advice you can use

to maintain the results . . . and enjoy that massage!

-OR-

Buy a whole new skin care regime at Sephora, or two very high-end, game-changing products, like Colbert MD Nutrify & Protect, $95, and Stimulate: The Serum, $135, my favorite splurges.

IF YOU HAVE $100 TO SPEND

Buy one new fabulous high-end treatment product.

-OR-

Stock up on a whole new regime at the drugstore. Brands to check out for high-tech at a low-price: Aveeno, Vichy, La Roche-Posay, Olay Professional Pro-X.

IF YOU HAVE $50 TO SPEND

Invest in a makeup primer that doubles as a sunscreen, like NARS Multi-Protect Primer SPF 30/PA+++, $32.

-OR-

Buy products for flare-ups and under-eye bags, and a spot pimple eraser or glycolic acid peel pads that will make you feel like you had a dermatological treatment again and again and again.

IF YOU HAVE $20 TO SPEND

Stock up on a supply of Greek yogurt and fresh berries for a skin-boosting breakfast.

-AND-

Buy a case of coconut water to hydrate from the inside.

-OR-

Make an at-home skin care emergency kit—Afrin for calming redness, uncoated aspirin for ridding pimples and ibuprofen for depuffing eyes, shrinking pimples, and preventing the damage from sun exposure.

-AND-

Buy a drugstore cooling eye wand like Garnier Nutritioniste Skin Renew Anti-Puff Eye Roller, $12.99. Store it in the fridge for added anti-puff power.

SKIN THAT MAKES YOU
LOOK LIKE

You Don't Have a Dime

- Shine that's more greasy than gorgeous

- Dry, flaky patches

- Large visible pores

- Blackheads

- Uneven texture

- Under-eye circles that make you look tired

- Too much Botox and fillers, signs of a dermatologist addiction

- Skin so peeled you look like a dried prune

- Premature aging (e.g., wrinkles, sunspots)

- Too much makeup covering your skin up (We'll get to that next!)

SKIN THAT MAKES YOU
LOOK LIKE

A Million Bucks

- Dewy glow

- Clear, clean complexion

- Skin that's alive, energized

- Even tone

- Smooth texture

- Bright

- Moisture-balanced—not too dry or too oily

- Soft and touchable

- Skin that looks poreless

- Luminescence

- Naturally flushed

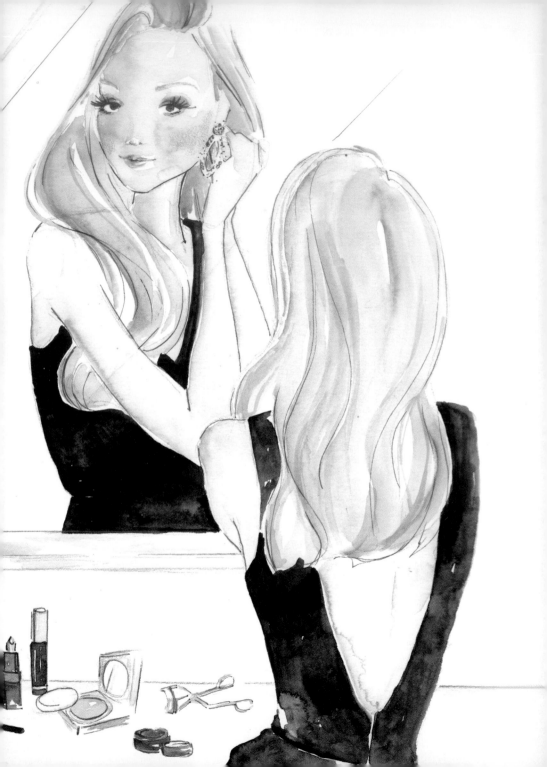

4

Expensive-Looking Makeup

You, Only Better

Have you ever noticed A-list actresses rarely make drastic changes to their makeup? Maybe they switch up their lipsticks, or wear new eye shadows, but you hardly notice because they look like themselves, only better. I call this "You, Only Better, Makeup," and it always looks expensive because it trumps all trends, is always appropriate, and never looks overdone. A key component of the look is that it's not the makeup that draws your eye, but the person wearing it. You focus on your favorite star's sparkle, her gorgeousness, the Harry Winston loaner necklace draped around her neck, not her eye shadow or blush. And that, my dears, is what expensive makeup is all about. It almost fades into the background, bringing out your beauty to make you the star, not your makeup. It has that "je ne sais quoi" quality you see on models in magazines, a glow that looks like it's more than skin-deep. It can be fashionable, but in a classic, not trendy, way—for instance, using the season's hottest eye color as a subtle accent, dabbed over a neutral shadow in the center of your lid, rather than as a strong overall eye statement.

The New Luminous Makeup Look

So what makes expensive makeup look so chic? Of course the way you apply it, and I'll give you plenty of new, upscale techniques. But it also has a lot to do with the products themselves. Cosmetics have gone through their own tech revolution, and opaque, heavy makeup is as much a dinosaur as the original iPad. With nanopigments, light-reflective spheres, and other innovations that make makeup more sheer, more radiant, and more spreadable (i.e., so easy to apply, you can often use your fingers!), makeup formulations keep getting better and better. And because of this, a luxurious new makeup look has evolved that is more about enhancing your features than hiding your flaws. This means if you haven't bought new makeup in a while, you're at a disadvantage—like using a computer from five years ago, you might want to consider a product update.

But here's some good news: You don't have to go for broke to do it. Technology trickles down to the masses pretty quickly and there are lots of great options at every price point. Which brings me to the eternal beauty question women ask me all the time . . .

A luxurious new makeup look has evolved that is more about enhancing your features than hiding your flaws.

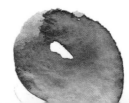

Is Expensive Makeup Worth It?

I can't say no but I can't say yes. It's a personal choice. Sometimes a Dior compact is the little luxury that lifts your mood and lets you indulge without taking out a loan. I think the best strategy is to mix it up. I've seen plenty of ritzy rich girls making up in the bathroom using Estée Lauder mascara and Revlon lipstick. It's like pairing a fashion find from Target with your favorite designer labels. You get a more individualistic look, not to mention cash to save or spend elsewhere.

Personally, I have to confess to a love of certain high-end products that I can't live without, but I also wear L'Oréal Paris, Physicians Formula, and Revlon, as well as a cool, smallish makeup brand called Milani, which you can find at Walgreens and Rite Aid, that seems to emulate some of my favorite high-end products. In fact, I have a second makeup bag for when I travel and go to the gym that's filled with inexpensive versions of many of my favorite high-end products. On my face, you can't tell the difference. The take away? More important than the cash you lay out is knowing where to skimp and where to save and what to do with each product.

I've seen plenty of ritzy rich girls making up in the bathroom using Estée Lauder mascara and Revlon lipstick.

The Four Rules of Modern Makeup

1 **Makeup should enhance instead of hide.** Focus on highlighting your features, rather than covering up your flaws.

2 **Less is more.** What you leave off is just as important as what you put on.

3 **Makeup should never overpower your features.** Your eye shadow, for example, should enhance your eyes, not distract from them.

4 **Color cosmetics should look like they come from within your skin** (not like they are sitting on top). "Using creams instead of powders gives skin a transparency that leaves the face looking juicy and full of life," says celebrity makeup artist Vanessa Scali.

GET YOUR MAKEUP DONE FOR LESS

(Or Even for Free)

Did you know that at most makeup counters—especially those in smaller specialty department stores like Barneys in New York—you can ask a makeup artist to do your makeup for a discreet tip? Lots of New York women do this after work to glam up for evening social events. At New York's Bergdorf Goodman, one infamous woman actually has a standing 5 P.M. appointment three times a week! That's a little much, but this is a great trick to know about when you want to look great for a party, a job interview, or just because you're wearing an old dress to an event and want to feel fresh and new. Space NK stores and many other smaller makeup boutiques offer complimentary makeup application at all times. The trick to getting out scot-free at any cosmetic counter is avoiding the temptation to take "just the lipstick," unless you love it and really want to buy it. You can ask for a Q-tip's worth wrapped in a tissue to touch up later. At some Sephoras and at all M•A•C counters you can get your makeup done for a $50 fee, redeemable in products. In either situation, the trick is to find a beauty advisor whose style you relate to and give them a try—you can always wash it off!

The Secrets Behind Expensive Makeup

Start a tear-sheet library of makeup looks you love—that's how beauty editors shape their stories and discover trends—and be on the lookout for the following features that define expensive makeup:

- **Makeup colors that match the natural colors in your skin,** lips, cheeks, the flecks of your irises, or even in the highlights of your hair: These look more expensive because they don't look artificial. Flip through a fashion magazine and you'll notice most celebrities stick to shades that look like they could be an enhanced version of their natural lip/skin color.

- **Sheer foundation or no foundation at all:** This gives a freshness and modernity to your look. "The minute you take away all that foundation and let your skin show, your makeup looks instantly chicer," says famed makeup artist Jeanine Lobell, who glams up Natalie Portman for her close-ups.

- **Expensive-looking makeup means attention to detail:** The blending away of demarcation lines and jagged edges, what my celebrity makeup artist friend and fellow chai-lover Jeffrey Paul calls "good tailoring." You'll never see a blob of color where the makeup starts and ends.

- **Makeup is sexier and more youthful when it looks lived-in:** Never messy, but not too perfect. Perfect looks contrived and robotic.

Makeup is sexier and more youthful when it looks lived-in.

Editing Your Makeup Wardrobe

One way to get the most bang for your buck with your cosmetic purchases is to be really stringent about what you buy. Start by cleaning out your makeup "graveyard," all the products you've bought but never use and can't bare to throw out for some reason. Give unused products to a homeless shelter or if you're really ambitious, sell them on eBay or swap them on MakeupAlley.com. Only save what looks good on you, what you use or love—makeup clutter is distracting, and it's so much easier to work from an edited collection.

Now it's time to see what's left and what pieces you might want to think about acquiring. In this chapter I'll give you lots of great choices whatever your budget in the hopes of helping you avoid blowing your beauty budget on bloopers. When you shop, use restraint; if you like high-end makeup, limit yourself to adding one or two luxury cosmetic items to your "wardrobe" the way you'd add designer clothes to your closet—think classic, not trendy. Add more as your budget and needs permit. And if you just have to have an übertrendy item, buy an inexpensive, "disposable" version. It also pays to be an educated consumer. Read product reviews online (MakeupAlley.com, Sephora.com, Amazon.com, or individual cosmetic company sites); your consumer peers are brutally honest and often a great source of try-before-you-buy advice.

Limit yourself to adding one or two luxury cosmetic items to your "wardrobe" the way you'd add designer clothes to your closet—think classic, not trendy.

THE TWENTY-ONE MAKEUP ESSENTIALS

TWO FOUNDATIONS
You can get away with one but need no more than two, a powder and a liquid, or one that's sheer and one with more coverage.

TWO CONCEALERS
A skin-matching or correcting one and a brightener/illuminating concealer (You can also get away with just the former and use foundation as concealer if you need more coverage.)

ONE POWDER
A brightening or translucent powder (Pressed is easier to use and store.)

TWO BLUSH SHADES
One tawny pink (neutral pink-brown) and one brighter shade (I prefer creams.)

ONE HIGHLIGHTER
A sheer pearly cream

FOUR EYE SHADOWS
A taupe and deeper neutral and a light gray and a deeper charcoal. Or two multi-color compacts or palettes, one in the brown family and one in the gray family.

TWO EYELINERS
A softer brown or a deep gray and a black

TWO MASCARAS
A thinner everyday one and a more dramatic one for night

ONE LIP LINER
In a color that matches your natural lip color

FOUR LIP PRODUCTS
A neutral, a pink, a red, and a gloss (How you apply lipstick can alter the intensity, negating the need for more colors.)

YOUR EDITED BRUSH COLLECTION

Makeup artists have piles of brushes, but you need no more than six, maybe even less, and they don't need to be expensive. I love Sonia Kashuk's affordable brushes from Target, Essence of Beauty brushes from CVS, and EcoTools natural bamboo brushes sold at many drugstores or online. You can also find all these brush shapes at an art supply store for a lot less money than the makeup counter, often with the same fancy mink and sable bristles or high-quality synthetics for half the price.

FOUNDATION BRUSH

A tapered brush to use with cream makeup.
I'm addicted to mine.

BLUSH BRUSH

A small fluffy one or duo-fiber brush,
not the tapered eighties kind that made your
blush look streaky.

CONCEALER BRUSH

Stiff, rounded, and tiny to dab
away breakouts without looking obvious.

EYE SHADOW BRUSH

Medium or small: It should fit easily
onto your lid for shadow application.
You can do without a crease brush by using
the tip of your shadow brush to blend shadow
in your creases.

EYELINER BRUSH

Either small, stiff, and rounded for gel or
cream liner application, or thin and stiff for
powder or gel/cream shadow lining.

BROW BRUSH

Skinny and stiff to fill in sparse brows
with miniature brow hair.

BETTER THAN BRUSHES

Honestly, many of my makeup brushes have become superfluous since I've switched to cream makeup formulas. These are the new tools makeup artists use to get luxe and luminous makeup:

Fingertips!

Finger-painting has become the go-to way to put on makeup. Makeup artists use their fingertips to apply and blend makeup for a more natural effect—that idealized expensive makeup look that appears to come from within your skin instead of sitting on top of it. Even if you use powder makeup, makeup pros suggest pressing it in with your fingertips—the heat will help it mesh with skin and look more like a part of it instead of a layer on top.

Built-in Brush Applicators

With brush-on foundation, where the product comes out of the brush itself, you no longer need a foundation brush. I also use the smudging end of an eyeliner as a liner brush with cream or powder shadow. Today's built-in brushes are a far cry from those old stiff brushes that came with powder blush and tended to shed.

The Beautyblender Sponge

Backstage at fashion shows, you'll always spot the signature pink Beautyblender sponge, a latex-free, ergonomically designed, non-disposable sponge used to get a professional blending effect in seconds. Its pointy tip and rounded, edgeless shape fits into facial contours and nooks and crannies like the sides of your nose to even out foundation and blend blush. I even use the tip to go over eyeliner and eye shadow to make them look smoother. Knockoffs I've seen work pretty well, too.

Wittled-down Q-tips

Makeup artists take the extra cotton off and twirl what remains around the tip to create a disposable "brush" to line and blend eyes and lips, or to apply lipstick. Or buy pointy cosmetic-applicator cotton swabs to use and toss.

Face Makeup Glossary

Skin is probably the most important aspect of today's expensive makeup look. Here's what you'll need to turn yours into one of your best features.

FOUNDATION—The new foundations work by adding a sheer luminosity to skin that adds some coverage, but not too much, to leave skin looking radiant. There are lots of formats to choose from; I personally like the new liquids that come with their own attached foundation brush (the product squirts through the brush). I also like baked powder foundations that react with your skin's natural oils when you brush them on to give you the luminous finish of a liquid with the ease of a powder. (Often mineral-based, they're not the old-school powder foundations that are fine for oily skin but otherwise too drying.)

Choosing a color: Most makeup artists believe it's best to match your jawline or even to apply the foundation right to your cheek—it should blend in and cancel out any redness or pinkness in your skin. New York City makeup artist Paul Podlucky thinks it's best to go a shade or two darker than your skin for a richer look. Alternatively, you can match your skin and warm it up with a few drops of a deeper-toned makeup pigment or a light dusting of a darker pressed powder. If you buy foundation at Sephora or a department store, ask

MY FAVORITE FOUNDATIONS

L'Oréal Paris True Match Super-Blendable Makeup, $10.95; L'Oréal Paris Visible Lift Smooth Absolute, $15.95; Milani Glow Natural Brush-On Liquid Makeup, $8.99, and Milani Even-Touch Powder Foundation, $8.49

SPLURGE

VIP Expert by Terry Liquid Foundation, $48; NARS Sheer Glow Foundation, $42; Bobbi Brown Moisture Rich Foundation SPF 15, $46; Laura Geller Balance-n-Brighten Baked Color Correcting Foundation, $31

MY FAVORITE PRIMERS

SAVE

E.L.F. Studio Mineral Face Primer, $6; L'Oréal Paris Studio Secrets Professional Magic Perfecting Base Face Primer, $12.95

SPLURGE

Embryolisse Lait-Crème Concentrè (24-Hour Miracle Cream), $25 (A three-in-one primer/moisturizer/makeup remover makeup artists swear by); NARS Multi-Protect Primer SPF 30/PA+++, $32 (If I'm going to spend money on a primer and add an extra step, it might as well have dual benefits!); Laura Geller Spackle Under Make-up Primer, $25 for a sample or have it applied and wear it for the day and see how you like it a few hours later.

MY FAVORITE TINTED MOISTURIZERS

SAVE

Sonia Kashuk Radiant Tinted Moisturizer SPF 15, $13.69; Boots No7 Soft & Sheer Tinted Moisturizer, $11.99; CoverGirl CG Smoothers SPF 15 Tinted Moisturizer, $8.50; Aveeno Positively Radiant Tinted Moisturizer SPF 30, $14.99

SPLURGE

Josie Maran Argan Tinted Moisturizer, $38; Tarte Smooth Operator Amazonian Clay Tinted Moisturizer with SPF 20, $36; NARS Pure Radiant Tinted Moisturizer SPF 30, $42; Glo Minerals Sheer Tint Base, $33.50

PRIMER—Makeup artists use a primer under makeup to even out skin and give your makeup products something to cling to—kind of like dry-coating a wall before you paint it. Most primers

also help sop up natural oil so it doesn't dissolve your makeup. They also invisibly improve the look of your skin (through light-enhancers) or block out redness so you need less opaque coverage on top. To save money, use the same primer to prime your eyelids for eye makeup and your lips for lipstick—it'll help makeup last without creasing or fading.

TINTED MOISTURIZER—The newest tinted moisturizers are more like a cross between moisturizer and foundation. They give a hydrated, luminous look with just enough coverage to even your skin out without looking like makeup.

BRIGHTENER—This is a new category of products previously used only by professionals that can replace your concealer or add sheen for a luminous look. Yves Saint Laurent's famous Touche Éclat, which now comes in a variety of shades and is a staple in every

MY FAVORITE BRIGHTENERS

SAVE

Physicians Formula Mineral Wear Talc-Free Mineral Correcting Concealer, $8.95; Sephora Collection Smoothing & Brightening Concealer, $14; Milani HD Advanced Concealer, $8.49; Boots No7 Radiant Glow Concealer, $12.99

SPLURGE

Yves Saint Laurent Touche Éclat, $40; Estée Lauder Ideal Light Brush-on Illuminator, $26.50; Make Up For Ever Professional HD Invisible Cover Concealer, $28; Benefit Cosmetics Erase Paste Brightening Camouflage for Eyes and Face, $26

makeup artists' kit, is the classic brightener. Instead of covering a flaw, say, under-eye circles, brighteners color correct and brighten up the area. Depending on your coloring, you'd use a pink brightener (for fair skin), yellow (for medium skin tones), or apricot (for olive and darker skin tones).

CONCEALER—Concealers are more useful for covering blemishes than dark circles, which are better eradicated with a brightener. Choose one that matches your skin and dab it on pimples one by one with small, painterly strokes to make them disappear without covering your whole face in base.

MY FAVORITE CONCEALERS

SAVE

Revlon PhotoReady Concealer, $10.99; L'Oréal Paris True Match Super Blendable Concealer, $8.95

SPLURGE

M•A•C Studio Finish SPF 35 Concealer, $17; Burberry Sheer Luminous Concealer, $40; Kevyn Aucoin Beauty the Sensual Skin Enhancer, $45

POWDER—Forget the old-school loose powder that made your skin look caked. The newer powders have light-reflection or

MY FAVORITE POWDERS

SAVE

Physicians Formula Virtual Face Powder Multi-Reflective Face Powder, $10.95; CoverGirl Clean Pressed Powder, $6.99

SPLURGE

Estée Lauder Lucidity Translucent Pressed Powder, $27; Koh Gen Do Maifanshi Natural Lighting Powder, $42; Glo Minerals Perfecting Powder, $34.50

brightening properties to add luminosity. If you get shiny in the T-zone, a translucent pressed powder applied just there will give you grease control without taking away glow. Top makeup artists use much less powder than they used to, preferring to blot away oil with a blotting paper and/ or applying powder after they've done all makeup, so as to see where it's really needed and therefore use less.

BLUSH—Creams or powders?

I prefer creams because they blend in and look like they come from within your skin. Plus the sheerness makes colors more universal, so it's harder to make a mistake and choose the wrong shade. Shimmer in a blush also helps make it more foolproof as the light-reflective particles in the product cancel out any harsh edges. "Look for a color that mimics the flush you'd get when you run up a flight of stairs," says makeup artist Vanessa Scali, who recommends Revlon Cream Blush in Berry Flirtatious for all skin tones. Have a brighter blush shade handy for days when you need a lift. (I'd swear my own bright blush was laced with antidepressants!) I find cream blush in a coral shade to be the most universal instant "happiness" shade on women of all skin tones.

MY FAVORITE BLUSHES

Physicians Formula Happy Booster Glow & Mood Boosting Blush, $11.95; Revlon Cream Blush, $9.79; Maybelline New York Dream Bouncy Blush, $7.99; Sonia Kashuk Crème Blush, $9.99; CoverGirl and Olay Simply Ageless Sculpting Blush, $10.49; Revlon Cream Blush in Berry Flirtatious, $9.70

SPLURGE

NARS the Multiple in Orgasm (love!), $39; Stila Convertible Color in Poppy (another Scali fave), $25; Laura Mercier Crème Cheek Color, $22

BRONZER—Rather than using it as blush, which looks very old-school, use a bronzer to warm up your whole look by dusting or dabbing it only where the sun would hit—temples, forehead, down your nose—or apply it sparingly as contour beneath your cheekbones. Choose a matte bronzer or use a liquid bronzer (or even just a foundation a few shades darker than your skin instead). Be sure to blend well. You can use a bronzer year-round but only as described; the idea is to give you some color without making you look tan.

MY FAVORITES BRONZERS

SAVE

Milani Baked Bronzer, $8.99; NYX Cosmetics Tango with Bronzing Stix, $10

SPLURGE

Bobbi Brown Bronzing Powder, $35; M·A·C Bronzing Powder, $23; Chanel Soleil Tan de Chanel Sheer Illuminating Fluid, $48

HIGHLIGHTER / ILLUMINIZER— A shimmer product used

MY FAVORITE HIGHLIGHTERS/ ILLUMINIZERS

SAVE

E.L.F. Essential Shimmering Facial Whip, $1; Sonia Kashuk Super Sheer Shimmering Highlighter, $9.99

SPLURGE

Burberry Fresh Glow Luminous Fluid Base, $48; NARS Illuminator, $29; Smashbox Halo Highlighting Wand, $32

to enhance certain areas of the face—the tips of your cheekbones, center of nose, top of forehead, Cupid's bow of mouth, inner corners of eyes— to add a 3-D effect. I like creams because they become a part of your skin, look more natural, and are easier to control than powders. Liquid highlighters, often called illuminizers, are a new product that you can mix into your makeup or apply under it for an unreal glow that lights up your face.

The Makeup Gurus Share Tips for a Flawless Face

BOOK AN APPOINTMENT WITH...

TALIA SHOBROOK
The Monet of Makeup

British-born, New York–based makeup artist Talia Shobrook has a fine arts degree, but found canvases boring so she paints on people—celebrities and models, that is. She's the genius behind the insanely gorgeous makeup at Marchesa fashion shows and was the mastermind behind the late Amy Winehouse's iconic eyeliner look. One of the things I admire about Talia's work is her luminous face makeup. She thinks paying attention to your skin is what's going to make your face look expensive and that women need to adjust trends to fit their skin tone and style rather than using the wrong shades just because they're "in."

"The new makeup approach to skin should be more about highlighting and enhancing than camouflaging. Think of your face makeup like a bra: It's the foundation of your whole look, without it nothing else fits."
—Talia Shobrook

Talia's Pet Peeve
"I don't understand brown lipsticks, everyone looks bad in them, washed out. A nude has to have some sort of pink or orange in it to look pretty."

Talia's Cheap Trick
Stash a few pieces of baking parchment paper in your purse to use as blotting paper.

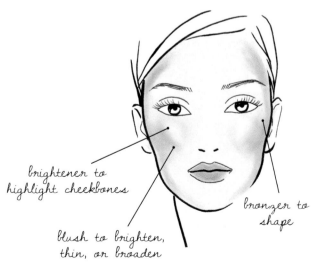

brightener to highlight cheekbones

bronzer to shape

blush to brighten, thin, or broaden

SIX STEPS TO A LUMINOUS FACE

by Talia Shobrook

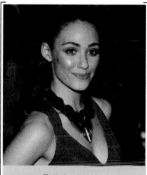

Talia's glow on
Emmy Rossum

1. APPLY SUNSCREEN
or primer. Talia prefers
sunscreen because besides
protecting your skin, it has a
sheen that exposes natural
highlights in your face that
you'll later enhance with
highlighter for even more
of a glow. She uses Vichy
and Avène sunscreens,
both well-priced European
brands sold at the drugstore.

**2. DILUTE YOUR
FOUNDATION** by adding
a little bit of moisturizer,
mixing the two on the back

of your hand (the heat of
your hand warms it up to aid
blending) before applying
it to your face. The combo
will give you a seamless,
rich, and hydrated finish that
blends easily into your skin.
You can then apply it with a
foundation brush, a sponge,
or your fingers (Talia uses
the Beautyblender.)

3. APPLY BRIGHTENER
to spots of your face you
want to highlight. The sheen
from the sunscreen will
guide you to where those
spots are on your face, but
essentially they're on the
tops of cheekbones, bridge
of nose, and Cupid's bow
above your lips. Choose the
color that works for your skin
(see brighteners in the Face
Makeup Glossary). To cover
stubborn dark circles or
flaws, mix a dab of foundation
with a dab of brightener to
create a luminescent cover-
up that won't look heavy.

4. APPLY BLUSH. Talia
actually uses lipstick as
blush but a cream blush
works, too. To broaden
your face, apply the blush
to the apple of your cheek
and blend outward. To thin
your face, apply the blush to
the apple of your cheek and
blend downward.

5. SHAPE YOUR FACE to
bring out your cheekbones
with a powder or cream
bronzer (without any
shimmer). Start underneath
the cheekbone, go up to
the temple almost into the
hairline, and then do the
same under the opposite
cheekbone, as if you were
creating a sideways
number 3.

**6. POWDER JUST THE
T-ZONE,** and only if you
need to.

Five Makeup Artist Secrets to Get Your Glow On

1 **Use highlighter** on your upper cheekbones for a rich-girl, candlelit effect, applying it with your index fingertip. You can also dab a bit onto the top of your brow bones. Use a pearly cream highlighter, a tiny bit of Vaseline, or even just your eye cream. To make your own highlighter, mix pearly white eye shadow with eye cream, Vaseline, or Weleda Skin Food, a makeup artist favorite (see page 145).

2 **Make your foundation look "airbrushed"** by spritzing your foundation brush with Evian Facial Spray or a moisturizing mist before using it. "It'll thin out your makeup and make it blend in easier and look more diffused," says makeup pro Bobby Wells, who taught me this trick.

3 **Apply a liquid illuminizer or shimmery moisturizer** over your regular moisturizer but underneath your base makeup. It'll make your skin glow like it does when you sit across a candlelit table. A NARS makeup artist showed me this trick and I get tons of skin compliments when I do it. Apply a dot to your forehead, one to your nose, one to each cheek and blend. You can also mix the illuminizer into your base makeup and apply it in one step. For a summery tanned look, use a more coral illuminizer, like NARS Illuminator in Orgasm (the so-called liquid orgasm!), or use a more pearly based illuminizer (like M·A·C Strobe Cream, Aveeno Positively Radiant Daily Moisturizer SPF 15, or Palmer's Skin Success Eventone Daily Skin Brightener with SPF 15) during the cooler months.

4 **Powder only the T-zone—forehead, nose, chin—**leaving natural shine under your eyes and on your cheeks.

5 **Spritz your finished makeup with a hydrating mineral or vitamin-infused water spray** (or even just tap water in a spray bottle!) like M·A·C Fix +, holding it about ten inches from your face, to give it a fresh, dewy radiance. "It will also take away any makeup-y chalkiness, smooth out foundation that's crept into fine lines, and thin down a too-heavy foundation application," says makeup artist Paul Podlucky. Let skin air-dry.

Your Expensive Eye Makeup Toolkit

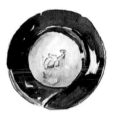

EYE SHADOW

Powder is classic but lately makeup artists and yours truly are using cream shadows to get a luminous look that'll blend into your skin more easily. Powders and creams both come individually or in duos, trios, or quads.

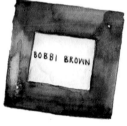

EYELINER

Available in pencils, gels, or liquids. The latter two will last longer, but most versions require a steady hand and a lining brush (some come with a brush) to avoid mistakes. I've found liquid liners that look like thin Sharpie markers to be the easiest to work with. The secret to applying any liner so it looks expensive is to pull the outer corner of your eye out with your forefinger to create a straight lining surface. You can layer a pencil under a shadow liner for staying power. Applying shadow on top—especially a shimmery one—can soften and diffuse uneven eyeliner edges and make mistakes undetectable. Sephora is a great place to find inexpensive, amazing eyeliners. I especially like their metallic ones.

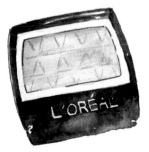

EYELASH CURLER

A must-have for makeup artists, the trick is to grab the lashes at the base and work the curler gently along the entire lash to create an even curl. When you hold the curl, pump it only slightly (heavy pumping can give them a step-up crease, kind of like the effect you get when you crease your hair with a curling iron—and just as tacky-looking).

MASCARA

You don't have to go expensive; most professional makeup artists actually swear by drugstore mascara. Use a natural-effect or thickening mascara for day—many artists prefer brown or brown-black (as opposed to jet-black) for a softer look. At night, go for a more dramatic "special effects" mascara. Or wear both at once: "I apply a volumizing formula from the root to the center of the lash and a lengthening formula from the center of the lash to the tips. The result is gorgeously lush and seductively lengthy lashes!" says makeup artist Vanessa Scali, who uses this trick on stars like Carrie Underwood, Christina Hendricks, and Ashley Greene.

DIY Expensive Eyes

The key to making your eye makeup look expensive is keeping a few of my rules of modern makeup in mind, specifically:

- **Less is always more.** (Go with a light touch, you can always add more.)

- **Makeup should never overpower.** (The goal is to enhance your eyes, not take them over.)

- **Makeup should look like it comes from within.** (Blend, blend, blend.)

And whether you buy high-end or low-end is up to you—in fact while most experts advise buying the best skin products money can buy, on eye makeup they often say it's okay to skimp.

EYE SHADOW KITS MADE EASY

To use singles: Depending on the depth of the shade, you can use it as a lid color, a crease/smoky-eye color, or a liner. Often one color of eye shadow is enough, pairing it with lots of mascara and little to no liner.

To use a duo: Use the lighter color on the lid itself, going up to but not above the crease, then use the darker color as liner. If the second color is a more medium than dark tone, you can use it to smoke out eyes by applying a little into the outer third of your crease, blending it down onto the outer corner of your lid.

To use a trio: Apply the medium color to the crease, blending it down on the lid, and the darkest color as liner to rim lids, then use the lightest color under the brow bone and/or at the inner corners.

To use a quad: Most four-color eye palettes can be applied like a trio; if it has two medium shades, one is probably for day, the other night. The darkest shade is meant to be used as a liner. And the lighter one again goes under the brow bone and/or at the inner corner.

CULT MASCARAS
MAKEUP ARTISTS SWEAR BY

For a natural daytime effect

SPLURGE

Bobbi Brown Everything Mascara, $24
Tarte Gifted Amazonian Clay Smart Mascara, $19
Trish McEvoy Lash Curling Mascara, $30
Lancôme Définicils, $25
Benefit They're Real! Mascara, $22

SAVE

Clinique Naturally Glossy Mascara, $15
L'Oréal Paris Double Extend Beauty Tubes Mascara, $10.95

For "special effect" drama
(i.e., false lashes in a tube!)

SPLURGE

Dior DiorShow Backstage Makeup Mascara $24.50
Lancôme Hypnôse Doll Lashes, $25, and L'Extrême, $25
Chanel Inimitable Intense Mascara, $30

SAVE

Maybelline New York Volum' Express the Falsies
Black Drama Waterproof Mascara, $7.77
Maybelline New York Lash Stiletto Voluptuous
Waterproof Mascara, $8.95
L'Oréal Paris Voluminous Original Mascara, $7.29
Rimmel London Sexy Curves Full Body Mascara, $7.49

Andrea's Everyday Expensive Eyes

(AND HOW TO VAMP THEM UP AT NIGHT)

I'm always asked how I get my eye makeup to look neutral, natural, and stylish at the same time. Here's my secret eye makeup technique.

1. EYE PRIMER. I start with a little foundation, concealer, or eye makeup primer on my lids to cancel out redness, absorb oil that would make the makeup fade, and give products I put on top something to grab on to. I rub it in from lid to brow.

2. CREAM SHADOW. I use a shimmer cream eye shadow in a taupe/grayish pinky/mauve color (sounds weird but looks very natural and pretty, kind of like skin!), applying it across my upper lids, then "V"-ing it up into my crease at the outer corner for depth, then blending it down toward my outer lashes using my fingers.

3. LINER. I line the top of my eyes with a pencil liner, often an automatic eyeliner (the self-sharpening kind, it slides on easier and gives a thinner line). I use an aubergine, an almost purply brown color, or a bronzey-brown, for the oomph of black without the harshness. If the line looks crooked or messy, I run the shimmer stick over it again to diffuse the edges. And on weekends, I often don't wear liner at all for a softer look.

When I'm particularly tired-looking and need a little more help than usual, I take advice I learned from makeup artist extraordinaire Bobbi Brown and add black liner on the outer third of each upper lash line, being sure it ends on an upward slant. Just a touch of black liner will lift your eyes up and distract from dark circles beneath them, truly! At night, I go more glam with

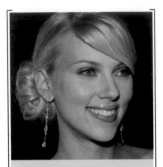

Scarlett Johansson's natural eye makeup says everyday expensive.

aubergine or brown
liner, just on top

primer from
lid to brow

taupe/mauve
shadow on "v"
and across
lash line

natural-looking
mascara

the black liner, applying it all the way across my upper lids from inner corner to outer corner, again extending it slightly out and up for an uplifting effect. Or I add a shimmery gunmetal cream shadow, applied with a liner brush, on top of my liner for pretty, sparkly definition

4. MASCARA. I like a kind of mascara called "tubing" mascara because it never runs and it comes off without leaving any darkness behind. It envelops your lashes with little tubes that wash off without eye makeup remover when you wash your face or take a shower. The Trish McEvoy and L'Oréal Paris mascaras I mentioned earlier on page 119 fall into this category, as does Clinique Naturally Glossy Mascara, $15.

WHAT I WEAR WITH IT!

I've got my makeup look down to a science, because as I've said, the idea is to look like myself, only better. Once I figured it out, I've stuck with it, switching up a product here and there for fun, to work with what I'm wearing, to go with a seasonal trend . . . or just because I feel like it! I use a brush-on foundation or, for a lighter look, a tinted foundation, then NARS the Multiple in Orgasm. (There's nothing like it, and I think every woman should own it!) on the apples of my cheeks, blending out to the sides; I dab a little more Orgasm around my hairline in tiny dots and blend it in to balance my face. I finish with lipstick—the good news is this eye is soft enough to work with any shade: red, plum, nude, or pink. For more specifics, take a peek at what's actually in my makeup kit—and duplicate products to get the look for less—on pages 141–143.

BOOK AN APPOINTMENT WITH...

ROMY SOLEIMANI

The Fashion Force

Romy Soleimani is a backstage friend whose incredibly expensive-looking makeup graces the faces of Liv Tyler, Diane Kruger, and Michelle Williams, as well as the models in many chic fashion shows and luxury editorial and advertising spreads. She has a great eye (as in great taste!) for makeup, and I especially love her signature evening eye makeup look. It's a little bit old Hollywood glam in a modern way but understated (not an easy combination to pull off!) and very sexy. And much copied by other celebrity makeup artists!

"Most women apply too much product at once. The key to expensive evening eye makeup is to apply sheer layers and work them into the skin for a more subtle effect."

—Romy Soleimani

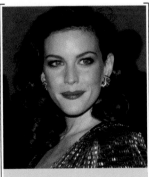

Romy's black-tie
eye on Liv Tyler

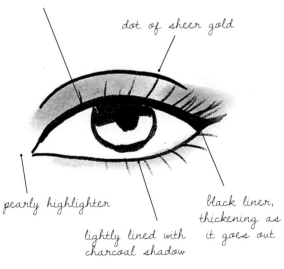

charcoal shadow
from lash line
to crease

dot of sheer gold

pearly highlighter

lightly lined with
charcoal shadow

black liner,
thickening as
it goes out

THE BLACK-TIE EYE

by Romy Soleimani

1. SHADOW. Apply a charcoal shimmery shadow on the lids up to the crease, winging it out a little bit. Then dot a sheer gold shimmer shadow right onto the middle of the lid, pressing it in to help it blend into the darker shadow and your skin.

2. UPPER LINER. Take a black pencil, or a powder or gel liner and apply it as close to the lash line as possible, thickening the line as you move to the outer corner and again winging it up a little at the end. Apply the charcoal shadow, this time as liner with a brush, over the black again, accentuating it into a bit of a cat-eye.

3. LOWER LINER. Dip a liner brush into the charcoal shimmery shadow, tap off the excess, then line the lower lash line with it to give it a sparkly allure without being a heavy black.

4. HIGHLIGHTER. Take a pearly, shimmery white cream highlighter, dip your pinky finger in it and pat it into the inner corners of your eye. Press it a few times to let the warmth of your finger blend it into your skin and become a glow.

5. MASCARA. Curl lashes and coat with an ultrablack (rich black) mascara. Romy uses CoverGirl LashBlast Length Mascara and L'Oréal Paris Voluminous Million Lashes Mascara in black.

6. LIPS. With eyes this dramatic, stay soft on lips and cheeks. "To keep it really elegant and sexy, use pinky nude blush and gloss," says Romi.

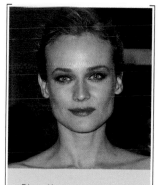

Diane Kruger wears it, too.

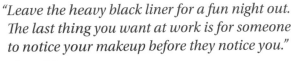

BOOK AN APPOINTMENT WITH...

LAURA GELLER

The Small-Screen Makeup Queen

Makeup artist Laura Geller of QVC fame has a makeup studio right near my apartment and did my wedding makeup. Here's her take on an eye that's good for work, no matter what your profession. It uses neutrals to enhance features without being too bold.

"Leave the heavy black liner for a fun night out. The last thing you want at work is for someone to notice your makeup before they notice you."

—Laura Geller

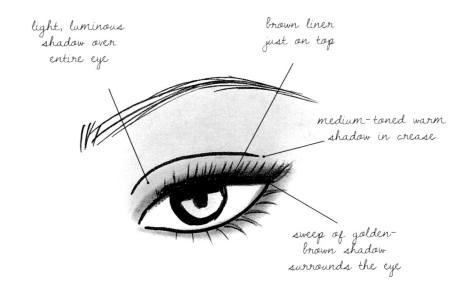

light, luminous shadow over entire eye

brown liner just on top

medium-toned warm shadow in crease

sweep of golden-brown shadow surrounds the eye

THE PROFESSIONAL EYE THAT GETS YOU PROMOTED

by Laura Geller

1. SHADOW. Lightly sweep a pale-toned luminescent shadow from lash line to brow bone.

2. LID AND CREASE. Dust a slightly deeper warm shadow—like the peach, pink, bronzy brown, and soft taupe combination in Laura Geller Baked Marble Eye Shadow Starburst, $23—onto lids and blend into the crease.

3. LINER. Apply a warm, golden copper-brown shadow into outer corner of eye and sweep it along the upper and lower lash lines for a soft liner look without any harsh edges, then apply a waterproof eyeliner in brown along the upper lash line to add definition but keep it soft.

4. MASCARA. Add volumizing black mascara for more eye emphasis.

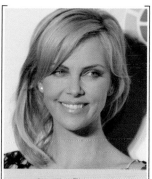

Charlize Theron in work-perfect eye makeup

PRO MAKEUP ARTIST SECRET: EYES FIRST, SKIN LAST

It started with skin in this chapter, but I want to point out that where you actually start your makeup application is debatable. Pro makeup artists begin with the eyes—and so do I—for two reasons. First, if you make a mistake and shadow, liner, or mascara ends up on your face, it's easier to wash off if you haven't put the rest of your makeup on yet. Second, going back to the less-is-more, enhance-instead-of-hide theory, once you've emphasized your eyes, you may not even notice flaws and will use less face makeup to cover them up! "Don't cover up, play up the good, and what's bad recedes," says my makeup artist friend Paul Podlucky, a guy whose work often appears on the chic well-dressed girls in *Vogue*'s party pages. "If you pull forth the eyes, put a nice cheek in there, apply lip color, and do a beautiful mascara, a lot of times things you think need to be concealed go away because you confuse people with the good stuff coming forth," he adds. Trust me, it's true.

BOOK AN APPOINTMENT WITH...

JEFFREY PAUL

The Beloved Makeup "Guru"

A spiritual guy who imparts his Eastern philosophy into his makeup artistry, Jeffrey likes to nurture his famous clients by bringing them chai and freshly cooked Indian food (as if making them look goddess-gorgeous wasn't enough!). You've seen his stunning smoky eyes, which always have a "dreamy" quality to them, on A-list celebrities walking countless red carpets. Sometimes they're dark and sultry, like smoke from a fire, created with dark charcoals and soft grays; other times they're soft and sensual, like a setting sun, achieved with soft golds and bronzes. Whatever the shade choice, the technique, which he shares here, stays the same. You can use this technique with a multitude of shadow colors, from nudes to mauves, browns to blacks.

"Smoky is more a makeup application method than a color. The idea behind it is that the colors fade out, one into the next."

—Jeffrey Paul

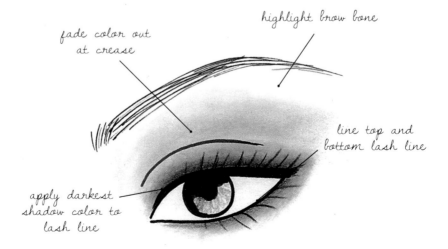

highlight brow bone

fade color out at crease

line top and bottom lash line

apply darkest shadow color to lash line

THE QUINTESSENTIAL SMOKY EYE

by Jeffrey Paul

1. PREP THE LID.
Begin a smoky eye with a base of primer, foundation, or concealer. The shadow will adhere to the moist underlayer and keep it vibrant and lasting longer.

2. RIM THE TOP AND BOTTOM
lash line with eyeliner. If you're going for a typical smoky eye with dramatic colors, start with a black, brown, or dark gray eyeliner. Use a liquid liner on top and a pencil on the bottom. This liner will be a base and enforce the technique of having the darkest colors in the center radiating outward as it gets lighter, much like smoke from a fire. Jeffrey then lifts the lashes and lines inside them, top and bottom, but don't try this at home without practicing first—as it's tricky to do and may be too dramatic depending on where you're going. I never do the inside liner thing (also called tight-lining)—it makes me feel queasy and look sleazy!

3. CHOOSE A SHADOW
color that is slightly lighter than your liner color, applying it across the lash line onto the lid with the color intensity strongest close to your lashes, blending up and fading out by the time you hit your crease. You can add a second slightly lighter shadow starting at the edge of the first one, blending it out to also fade at the crease.

4. HIGHLIGHT FROM THE ARCH
above the crease up to the brow bone using a skin tone or lighter shadow.

5. USE A CLEAN BLUSH
to blend powder shadow or a finger or cosmetic sponge to blend cream shadow, blurring away the edges so you get a gradation of color, from darkest at the lash line fading up to the brow bone.

6. ADD MORE LIQUID EYELINER
to the lash line if needed. Finish with several coats of mascara.

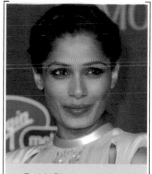

Freida Pinto's smoky eye looks chic not clubby.

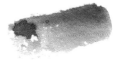

Expensive Eyeliner Looks

Eyeliner is a makeup item that can be your best friend or your worst enemy. Most women go wrong and break my modern makeup rules when they use the same eyeliner techniques they've had since high school—or try to copy a trendy look that ends up distracting from their eyes instead of enhancing them (for instance wearing Katy Perry eyeliner when you're not Katy Perry). Always remember, with eyeliner less is more and good taste is all about restraint and refusal (rule #1) and be sure your eyeliner doesn't overpower (rule #2). The best way to figure out what looks good on you is to experiment. Go to the makeup counter and let them do your eyes a few times and see what looks good and then adopt it into your repertoire with whatever makeup you use. Here are some questions and solutions to get you started.

> *Most women go wrong and break my modern makeup rules when they use the same eyeliner techniques they've had since high school.*

Do your eyes look good with liner all the way around, top and bottom?

Mine don't. It closes them up. I always adjust my liner by using a darker color across the top to lift them and usually leaving the bottom bare, but sometimes rimming them with a neutral taupe when I want more definition, say for photos, or using a light touch of mascara (Clinique's Bottom Lash Mascara, $10, is genius for this). Lining just the tops, by the way, gives your eyes a more awake, uplifted look. (And who couldn't use that?)

IS GLITTER EVER CHIC OR ALWAYS TACKY?

Sometimes you want a little special effect with your eye makeup and glitter seems like a great option. Talia Shobrook has it all figured out. She suggests using solid glitter shadow with tiny embedded glitter particles—it's less messy, and it won't get all over your face and look tacky. Dab it on with a finger and press it into the center of your lids over your shadow base color as a highlight. She likes the Ultimate Pearl Eye Shadow from NYX, a cult line of professional-quality cosmetics at drugstore prices (you can find it online, and at Ulta or Rite Aid for around $7).

I also love a makeup idea presented by M•A•C at the Jason Wu show a few years ago—M•A•C Pigment in Old Gold, $20, was lightly pressed onto the lids and worn with no liner and a little bit of mascara. The effect was like a burst of sunshine that brightened up the models' eyes, but was really only recognizable as glitter when they shut them. By the way, to keep glitter attractive and not glitzy, you want it to stay where you put it. Makeup artists catch straying glitter with a piece of scotch tape!

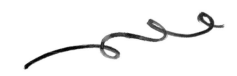

Do your eyes look good with liner that starts at the inner corner and works its way to the outer corner?

An alternative is to line just from above the pupil outward on just tops, or tops and bottoms (to create kind of a sideways *V*). This gives you a more wide-eyed effect.

Do your eyes look good with liner inside the rim line?

As I said in the smoky eye instructions, this is one of *my* pet peeves! It always runs and it looks like it might have hurt, not pretty. And even if you can do it without tearing up, it looks painful and artificial to everyone else. Yet women love the effect because they think it's sexy. I say if you do it, use waterproof liner, keep it light, and save it for night. Or trade your black for a softer gray or brown.

Do your eyes even need liner?

You don't have to wear it. Sometimes just focusing on making your lashes look amazing is enough. Makeup artist Talia Shobrook likes to dip an eyeliner brush into a thin mascara and use it at the very base of the lids like liner to emphasize the eyes invisibly (not glossy or matte like eyeliner, it just looks like you're wearing mascara). Using a taupe or brown shadow or pencil as a liner is another way to get a soft, natural look if you don't like or need a heavy line.

Blake Lively's Sexy Shimmer Liner Look

An incredibly easy alternative to traditional eyeliner, Blake's signature is a rim of glowy golden shimmer around her lids— instead of a harsh-colored liner. The look was created by her makeup artist Amy Tagliamonti on the set of *Gossip Girl*. (Amy once told me Blake would kill her if she shared it, but I dished on it in *Glamour* and will do it again here!)

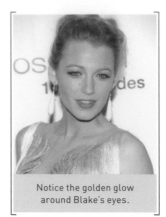

Notice the golden glow around Blake's eyes.

1 **Rim both tops and bottoms with a liner brush using a golden shimmer shadow,** like Stila Kitten or Oasis, sometimes applying an extra dot or a pearl-toned shimmer to the inner corners.

2 **Use a cream shimmer shadow with a brush or a shimmer stick,** blending it to avoid demarcation lines—it should just look like a diffused sparkle that surrounds your eyes— and makes them look as glowy as if they were candlelight.

FOUR LINER LOOKS THAT ALMOST ALWAYS LOOK CHEAP

- **Blue or green liner on blue or green eyes.** Too matchy-matchy! It actually distracts from your eye color instead of bringing it out. You're better off with a brown, taupe, charcoal, black, or plum.

- **Heavy black liner circling your lids** and/or applied to the inside rims of your upper and/or lower lids. I love Kate Middleton and the fact that she does her own makeup, but sometimes she's guilty of this one.

- **Liquid liner that looks messy.** If you can't apply it in a straight line, don't apply it. And keep to a thin, more subtle line when you use it during the day.

- **White liner in the inside rims.** It's supposed to make you look less sleepy but I think instead it looks really creepy! Try a skin-toned liner for a similar, but prettier wakeup-makeup effect.

Lashes

I don't know how it happened, but lashes have become such an obsession. You can't flip a magazine page or watch a television show without seeing at least one mascara advertisement. And with new technologies allowing for more long-lasting lash enhancers, like lash extensions, Latisse, and semipermanent mascaras, you can get great lashes that'll make wearing any other makeup almost unnecessary. But be careful—it's easy to go overboard and clumpy; spidery lashes that look stiff and untouchable are not doing you any favors. Want a prettier lash look? Here's how celebrity makeup artists use mascara to get gorgeous, clump-free lashes.

The Lush Mascara Application Technique

1 **Wipe the mascara wand off with a tissue** to remove excess. I like to use a tubing mascara because it never smudges. For more mascara choices, see cult celebrity mascaras, page 119.

2 **Comb through your lashes with the wand,** starting with the tip of the wand at the root of the lashes, wiggling up to the ends.

3 **For more intensity or if your lashes are light in color,** sandwich them by coating them on both sides.

4 **Before they dry, to remove excess, comb through lashes again with a disposable mascara wand** (you can buy them at beauty supply stores), mascara comb, or my choice, a toothbrush—the new flossing toothbrushes with different-size bristles are great.

Get the Look of Long, Luxurious Lash Extensions with Mascara

I love this tip from Talia Shobrook: Layer two drugstore mascaras, a thin natural-effect one and a heavier special-effect one. Apply the thin one to your lashes using the lush mascara application technique on the previous page, let dry, then use the special-effects mascara on the outer third of your lashes to fan them out and make them look long and flirty like extensions or false eyelashes . . . but not as fake. For an even more natural look, use one natural-looking mascara, the first coat all over, the second coat to flirt out the outer third of your lashes.

> *Layer two drugstore mascaras, a thin natural-effect one and a heavier special-effect one.*

Longer-Lasting Lash Options

Lash extensions

Women who do them are obsessed. Like hair extensions, lash extensions are tiny faux lashes applied to your lashes to give them extra length. Though they can cost a fortune, from $100 to $300 for the initial application and slightly less for touch-ups, some women say they change their life. The trick with lash extensions is to keep them looking as natural as possible. It's okay if they look like you're wearing mascara . . . what you don't want is for them to look like spiders—which plenty of them do! Having a half-set applied, or just getting them on the outer third of your lashes is less timely, costly, and looks more believable. You'll need to go back every three weeks or so for touch-ups. I prefer to get them before a vacation or at a time when I want to look great without fuss, but then I'll have them removed because they tend to look cheesy after a while when you keep touching them up.

Semipermanent Mascara

This is like long-lasting nail polish for your lashes. They're safe and pretty amazing, results last from two weeks (Cry Baby brand) to six weeks (LashDip) but they're not maintenance-free—you have to coat them with a special lash product or they get stiff and hard. Also great for vacation and/or allergy season, when you can't apply any eye makeup. (Get them done before the allergies start!)

Latisse and Lash-Growing Mascaras and Liners

Latisse is a prescribed cosmeceutical that grows your lashes. You apply it like eyeliner along your upper lash line at night. Some women are afraid of it because a very uncommon side effect is that it'll darken light eyes, but more commonly the problem is that if you don't apply it really carefully, you'll grow lashes in odd places and/or the lashes will stick out in funny directions. But friends of mine who use it—and the brand's celebrity endorsers, like Brooke Shields and Claire Danes—say it truly works and is a godsend, negating the need for mascara and giving you the look of lash extensions or false lashes that makes anything but lipstick unnecessary. The lash-growing mascaras you see advertised these days? Most use peptides, an ingredient used in skin care products to stimulate skin cell growth. Buy a drugstore version to test one out on the cheap.

How to Apply False Lashes Like a Pro

It's easier than you think, and celebrities and even princesses and their hot sisters have used this hidden enhancement to look amazing without having to apply too much makeup. Funny, but with false eyelashes you can actually look more natural because once your eyes really pop, you can use less makeup.

1. CUT A FALSE LASH STRIP in three as in sketch A. Use the outer third of the false lash on the outer third of your lashes for a super-enhanced look. For a softer, less obvious faux lash, use the inner third on the outer third of your lashes—they'll make lashes look thicker and fuller instead of longer and flirtier. Alternatively, use the middle section on its own, above your pupils, to make your eyes look larger.

2. USE BRUSH-ON CLEAR GLUE—from Ardell and sold at the drugstore, it's less drippy and messy than the kind that comes in tubes and becomes invisible on your eyes. You can also try lash adhesives—they have a sticker-like material on the edge so you don't need glue.

A

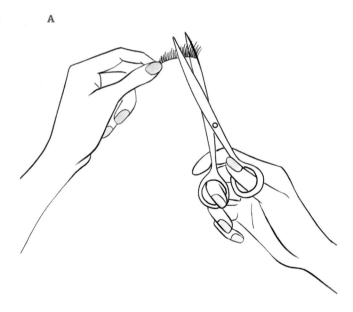

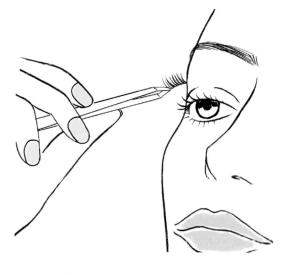

B

If you use the tube glue, buy black—if you apply too much, it'll disappear into the base of your lashes and is easily hidden with black liner.

3. HOLD THE PIECE OF LASH STRIP with a tweezer, apply glue to the edge, then apply it to your eye as in sketch B. You can then use the tweezers to hold it down until the glue dries. Note: Sephora makes a great lash-applying tool that works even better than tweezers.

4. USE BLACK GEL LINER across the top lash line if you need to hide the glue; if not, just a sweep of a soft shimmery champagne eye shadow is all you need for a clean, less-is-more eye look.

5. A BIT TRICKIER but more natural-looking are individual faux lashes. Celeb artists prefer the knot-free kind. You'll find a few options under the Cheap Secrets of Expensive Makeup Artists on page 144.

ALL FAKE EYELASHES ARE A CHEAP SECRET! It's all about finding ones that work for you and look natural. New York socialite and reality TV star Olivia Palermo, who is known for her rich-looking fashion and beauty aesthetic, told me Revlon Fantasy Lengths Maximum Wear Glue-On Eyelashes were her surprising eye makeup addiction when I interviewed her for *Glamour.* They're about $6 and have a self-adhesive sticky edge that negates the need for glue.

Brows

Brows frame your face and having the right shape is crucial (we'll get to that in the next chapter), but here I want to focus on brow makeup. You may not even need to bother with it—I rarely wear brow makeup during the day—but if and when you need some brow enhancement, the key is to go for the most natural-looking fill-in effect possible.

How to Fill in Your Brows So They Don't Look Fake

- **Use brow powder with a stiff brush instead of a pencil.** It's easier and more natural-looking. Los Angeles–based makeup artist and brow expert extraordinaire Brett Freedman has his own line of brow powders called Vanitymark that come in seven shades—including a great one for platinum blondes—and are used by a lot of celebrities. At $16, they last forever and are worth the investment for almost a custom-match brow product. If you do go with pencil, be sure it's a hard, thin one, not a thick, waxy one.

- **Go a little lighter than your natural brow shade with your fill-in color for the most believable look.** Brett Freedman applies this strategy when working with Catherine Zeta-Jones, using a soft brown instead of a deeper brown to match her brow hair. "If I used a darker brown to fill it in, it would match her hairs too closely and it would look too solid and drawn in," he says. Brunettes lighter than Catherine, brunettes with blonde highlights, and honey blondes should use a taupe color. For redheads, a soft beige-ginger is a good choice. The only exception to the go-lighter brow fill-in rule is if you're a very pale blonde, in which case going a shade darker brings out your brows and prevents them from disappearing.

HOW TO MASTER THE NUDE LIP

There's nothing more classic and chic than the perfect nude mouth—not too brown or too pink, not too glossy or too matte. But the right color is tricky to find. In fact, so many women cheapen their look with the wrong nude lipstick—it can drain all the color away from your face. To find your perfect nude, look for one that makes your face light up and look awake, not tired. It may take some swatching to find the right one, but if you have to question that it looks good on you, it probably doesn't. Here are some guidelines from Talia Shobrook to help you choose.

If your skin is light, go for a pinky nude like Burberry Lip Cover in Delicate Rose, $30; or NYX Cosmetics Matte Lipstick in Pale Pink, $6.

If your skin is medium, go for a nude that has both pink and orange in it like Burberry Lip Cover in English Rose, $30; or NYX Cosmetics Round Lipstick in Tea Rose, $4.

If your skin is dark, go for an orangey nude like NARS Lipstick in Honolulu Honey, $24; or NYX Cosmetics Round Lipstick in Pure Nude, $4.

• Create a more natural-looking brow by adding a few strokes of fill-in to the rest of your brows, even if you don't need it. Go lightly. Then use a "spooly," the end of the brow pencil that looks like a mascara brush, to blend. (You can also use a clean, old toothbrush!)

Lips

The good news about lipstick in the new makeup era is that it's easier to apply than ever. Many makeup artists now use their fingers or apply it straight from the tube instead of with that fancy little lip brush women pulled out of their purses in the eighties. Changing how you apply a lipstick also lets you get multiple looks from one color, which saves money. Lipliner has gotten a makeover, too, with most artists using only natural liner to give lips natural-looking definition, whatever the color they apply on top. Part of this has to do with the focus on eyes that I just told you about. With strong eyes, you need softer lips to avoid looking like a drag queen. And when I say softer, I'm referring not just to the texture but to the sharpness of the lip shape—neat but natural looks more expensive than a mouth with too precise or, worse, over-shaped edges.

Five Lipstick Mistakes That Cheapen Your Makeup and How to Avoid Them

1 **Too much gloss.** To avoid a goopy or X-rated look, apply a little gloss just to the centers of the mouth, use a less shiny balm instead of gloss for a more subtle sheen, or try one of the new lipstick gloss pencils, which offer color and definition with the perfect amount of not-too-glossy shine. I love NARS Velvet Gloss Lip Pencil, $24.

2 **Visible lip liner.** Ick. 'Nuf said. To avoid lips looking outlined, stick with a lip liner that matches your natural lip color no matter what shade of lipstick you wear—and apply it just to the parts of your mouth that need definition. See nude liner suggestions on the next page.

3 **Lipstick on your teeth.** To avoid walking the red carpet with lipstick-stained teeth, makeup artist Gita Bass has all her celeb clients use the old put-your-finger-in-your-mouth-and-take-it-out trick to get rid of excess lipstick that could migrate to your teeth.

4 **Applying lipstick over chapped or dry lips.** To avoid a flaky lip look, exfoliate your mouth first. And if it doesn't help, switch to a colored healing lip balm instead of lipstick (I like Burt's Bees Tinted Lip Balm, $7) for a soft, pretty lip look until your mouth heals—and play up your eyes!

5 **Plumping lips by applying lipstick or liner past the edges.** Another big no-no. To avoid a penciled-on lip augmentation look, use a light nude shimmery gloss on the center of your lips. It's a better way to add the illusion of volume without looking artificial.

DEMYSTIFYING THE RED LIP

Being able to pull off a red lip with style is a real coup. Once again, Talia Shobrook to the rescue!

Pick the perfect red. If your skin is light, go with a blue/red. If your skin is medium, go with an orange/red. If your skin is dark, go with a berry red.

Try Burberry Lip Cover in Union Red No.17, $30. "It's the most universal red. It works for all skin tones. It has a little bit of everything in it. I don't know how they do it but it looks great," says Talia. A great drugstore alternative is NYX Cosmetics Black Label Lipstick in Cherry, $7.50, or Target's Sonia Kashuk Velvety Matte Lip Crayon in Rosey Nude 10, $7.59.

Use a brightener (the kind I suggested as a new kind of concealer or see skin care glossary) all over the lips to block out the color and highlight the natural lip shape. You can also use a little bit of foundation or M·A·C Lip Erase, $18.50.

Smile. It's the easiest way to get a straighter application surface, and it tightens up your lips so that lipstick goes on in a smooth, even layer. Apply from the tube or, if using an intense hue, with a lip brush; soften the edges with a Q-tip.

How to Make Lips Look Luxe

1. START WITH SMOOTH LIPS. If yours are chapped or dry, use Vaseline or Aquaphor with a dry toothbrush to exfoliate them. Apply a lip primer or lip balm to create a smooth surface. Blot your lips with a tissue to take off any excess that would prevent lip color from adhering.

2. APPLY LIP COLOR, either straight from the tube or with your fingers, starting at the centers and blending outward for a more natural, voluptuous look. If you use a stain, a finger is definitely best because it'll look more natural and less painted on.

3. APPLY A LITTLE SHEEN or a lighter shimmery shade just to the centers of lips to make them look fuller. You want a little shine but not too much gloss.

4. (OPTIONAL) If you think your mouth needs more shape, use a little natural liner along the tops and bottom sides, leaving out the Cupid's bow and corners, and blending well to diffuse the line (like Spanx, invisible support you don't want to see!).

5. (OPTIONAL) DAB a pearly cream highlighter in a soft V-shape at the Cupid's bow.

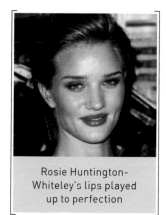

Rosie Huntington-Whiteley's lips played up to perfection

VANESSA SCALI'S MUST-HAVE LIP LINERS

I gave Vanessa Scali one of her first makeup jobs during my *Cosmo* days; now she's traveling the world with the stars of *Twilight* and making up actresses like America Ferrera and Christina Hendricks. These are the go-to shades she uses with any color lipstick to define her clients' mouths, without leaving any evidence that they're even there:

Rimmel London Exaggerate Automatic Lip Liner in Addiction, $5.79; Lancôme Le Lipstique in Bronzelle, $24.50; M•A•C Lip Pencil in Spice, $14

add sheen to fill out lips

keep color soft at the corners

BLUE-CHIP LIPSTICKS:
THE TOP TEN LUXE LIP SHADES MAKEUP ARTISTS SWEAR BY

There are some lipsticks that are like blue-chip stocks: good investments. These ten shades fall into that category and are the lipstick equivalent to Google, Apple, GE, and AT&T. I hear about them again and again at fashion shows and when artists tell me what they've used on celebrities.

1
NARS Dolce Vita Lipstick: The perfect, deep rosy pink neutral

2
NARS Jungle Red Lipstick: The perfect true red

3
M·A·C Lipstick in Ruby Woo: The perfect retro red

4
Chanel Rouge Allure Satin Lip Colour in Lover: A classic blue-toned red

5
Chanel Rouge Coco Hydrating Crème Lip Colour in Paris: A bright red with a tint of pink

6
Chanel Rouge Coco Hydrating Crème Lip Colour in Gabrielle: A creamy vintage-inspired red

7
M·A·C Viva Glam II: A twist on a classic nude with pink and mauve undertones

8
Bobbi Brown Lip Color in Pink: The quintessential baby-doll pink

9
Tom Ford in Casablanca: A deep rosy pink

10
Clé de Peau Beauté Extra Rich Lipstick in R5: A deep pink with coral undertones

What's in My Makeup Bag?

I did an experiment and was pleasantly surprised that I could duplicate all my makeup at the drugstore for less than a third of the total price. Here are the two versions. I now keep the less expensive one in my work/gym/travel bag and the expensive one at home. Give it a try yourself—google your favorite products with the words "drugstore version" or "duplicate" and you may find a gold mine of suggestions from other women who've already done the research.

TINTED MOISTURIZER

Andrea's Kit: NARS Pure Radiant Tinted Moisturizer SPF 30, $42
Duplicate Kit: Sonia Kashuk Radiant Tinted Moisturizer SPF 15, $13.69

FOUNDATION

Andrea's Kit: VIP Expert by Terry Light - Expert, $48
Duplicate Kit: L'Oréal Paris Visible Lift Smooth Absolute, $15.95

CREAM BLUSH

Andrea's Kit: NARS the Multiple in Orgasm, $39
Duplicate Kit: NYX Cosmetics Tango with Bronzing Stix in Merengue Flush, $10

MASCARA

Andrea's Kit: Trish McEvoy High Volume Mascara in Jet Black, $30
Duplicate Kit: Clinique Lash Power Mascara, $14.50

EYELINER

Andrea's Kit #1: Chanel Paris Stylo Yeux Waterproof Long-Lasting Eyeliner in Cassis, $30

Duplicate Kit #1: New York Color Waterproof Eyeliner Pencil in Smokey Plum, $3.99

Andrea's Kit #2: By Terry Ligne Blackstar Intense Liquid Eyeliner in Black Friction, $43
Duplicate Kit #2: NYX Cosmetics Super Skinny Eye Marker in Carbon Black, $9

Andrea's Kit #3: By Terry Crayon Khol Terrybly in Brown Stellar, $33
Duplicate Kit #3: Sephora Collection Liner Electro in Choc Electro, $8

EYE SHADOW

Andrea's Kit #1: By Terry Ombre Blackstar in Blond Opal, $42.50
Duplicate Kit #1: Sephora Collection Crayon Jumbo Liner 12HR Wear in Taupe, $10

Andrea's Kit #2: By Terry Ombre Blackstar in Black Pearl, $42.50
Duplicate Kit #2: Sephora Collection Crayon Jumbo Liner 12HR Wear in Gray, $10

Andrea's Kit #3: By Terry Ombre Blackstar in Misty Rock, $42.50
Duplicate Kit #3: Jemma Kidd Makeup School Stardust Crème Shadow in Comet, $18

POWDER BLUSH/CONTOUR

Andrea's Kit: NARS Powder Blush in Douceur, $27
Duplicate Kit: Maybelline New York FIT Me Blush in Deep Coral, $5.51

POWDER

Andrea's Kit: Laura Geller Balance-n-Brighten Baked Color Correcting Foundation, $35
Duplicate Kit: Milani Minerals Compact Makeup, $8.99

LIP COLOR

Andrea's Kit #1: NARS Velvet Gloss Lip Pencil in New Lover, $24
Duplicate Kit #1: Sephora Collection Ultra Vinyl Lip Pencil in Gorgeous Peach, $12

Andrea's Kit #2: Laura Mercier Crème Lip Colour in Audrey, $22
Duplicate Kit #2: Sephora Collection Rouge Cream Lipstick in Decollete, $12

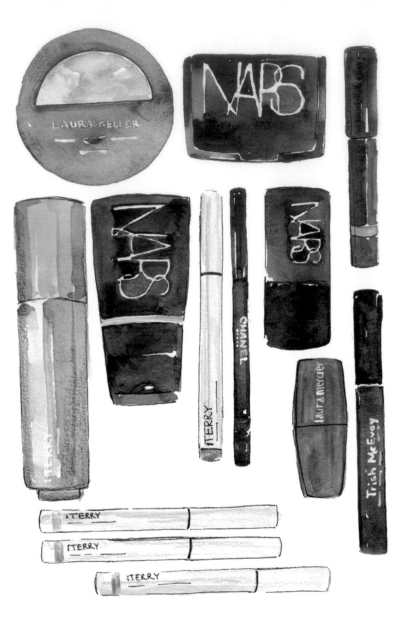

ANDREA'S MAKEUP KIT TOTAL COST: $500.50

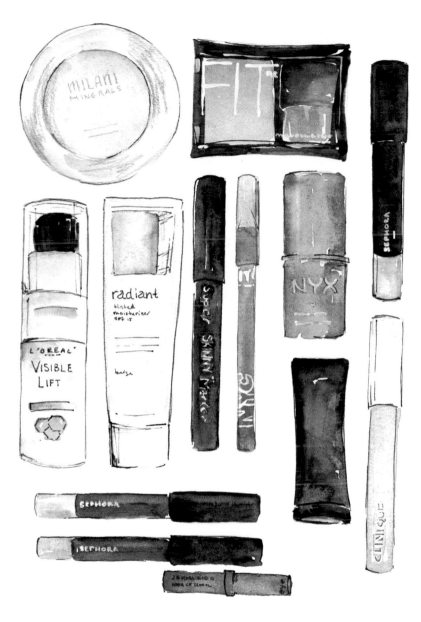

DUPLICATE MAKEUP KIT TOTAL COST: $151.63

The Cheap Secrets of Expensive Makeup Artists

L'Oréal Paris Voluminous Original Mascara

Makeup artists agree that it works as well if not better than any high-end mascara. It's a tubing mascara that works by forming little tubes around the lashes that come off easily without eye makeup remover when you wash your face.

Maybelline Lash Discovery Mascara

Rose-Marie Swift, the queen of supermodel makeup, whose client list includes the likes of Miranda Kerr and Gisele Bündchen, says a wand makes the mascara and this one is flawless. It lets you get every single lash.

Powder Puffs and Cotton Swabs

Rose-Marie Swift points out that these drugstore classics are a must-have for a complete makeup kit. Useful for everything from removing makeup mistakes to smudging eyeliner, a pointed cotton swab even makes a great disposable eye-lining brush. Swift recommends looking for synthetic-free 100 percent cotton versions.

Nivea Tinted Lip Balm, A Kiss of Cherry

Romy Soleimani loves this cherry red lip tint/balm. "It makes your lips baby soft. The slip is perfect, it doesn't collect anywhere, it's not too berry, just a gorgeous cherry that looks good on everyone. It's great-looking, like a YSL color," she says.

Ardell Duralash Natural in Short Brown

A favorite of makeup artist Nick Barose, who says he loves how natural these individual lashes look. Barose adds three to five of them to the outer corner of upper eyes to give them a lift.

L'Oréal Paris True Match Super Blendable Makeup and True Match Concealer

I've heard makeup artists rave about this product—even makeup artists who work for other prestige brands love it. I found my perfect shade on the first try—I bought an N shade for neutral even though I'm a warm—neutrals are more mistake-proof, and they cancel out redness and blend right in.

Cetaphil Moisturizing Lotion

Another oldie-but-goodie. Makeup artist Kim Bower uses it on a Q-tip or cotton ball as a mistake eraser and loves the moist, non-greasy texture it gives skin after cleansing, which is a great base for makeup.

L'Oréal Paris Studio Secrets Professional Color Smokes Eye Shadow in Blackened Smokes

A favorite of makeup artist Jeffrey Paul, it's got the same colors as some of his high-end expensive designer palettes... for $5.99!

Essence of Beauty Synthetic Foundation and Powder Brush

"This brush from CVS is one of the softest foundation brushes I've used and it never sheds," says makeup artist Kelsey Deenihan. I like the six-brush set, it covers all your brush needs for less than $10.

CoverGirl Eye Enhancers 1-Kit Shadow in Swiss Chocolate

"It's the perfect brown. It doesn't have too much red in it, it's not too dark. It's the perfect contrast to bring out the blue in blue eyes and it's a great eye contour shade for women of color," Viola Davis's makeup artist Autumn Moultrie told me.

Colorganics Hemp Organics Lip Tints

Romy Soleimani also loves the reds and berry tones of these sheer lip colors—they're completely organic and gorgeous, and cost just $3.99 each. Wahoo!

Weleda Skin Food

I spotted this once in Romy's bag and found out she uses it for everything— as a body highlighter to add a glossy look on editorial photo shoots, to mix in with drugstore shimmer shadow to create a shimmery cream highlighter to use on hot spots like collarbones, top of shoulders, lips, eyes, and tips of cheekbones.

CoverGirl Outlast Lipstain and Revlon Just Bitten Lipstain + Balm

"I use these lip markers as a base under lipstick. They're great, especially for a long night out because they really last," says Romy.

Albolene Moisturizing Cleanser, Unscented

This oldie-but-goodie product takes off makeup easily and gently, leaving skin hydrated instead of dry like other makeup removers.

Couturize Your Makeup

PARK AVENUE PRETTY

At work: Clean-cut and professional—light foundation, radiant pink cheeks, precise dark brown liner, lips moistened with a tinted lip balm, and you're good to go.

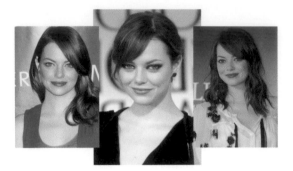

At night: Go for thin black liner and lots of mascara or a bronze shimmer shadow rimming your lids. Add a pop of pink blush with flecks of gold to the apples of cheeks and a rosy or coral shimmery lip pencil or gloss.

On the weekend: Wear tinted moisturizer with SPF, a touch of rosy blush, brown mascara, and a lip gloss or tinted lip balm that brightens your face. Polished, but casual. **Think:** *Emma Stone*

HOLLYWOOD BOHO

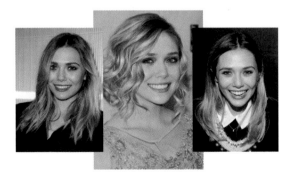

At night: Wear understated cat-eye black liner or a charcoal shimmer liner, with soft pink blush and pale nude lips. Or pair a neutral shimmer on your eyes with plenty of mascara and a trendy lip shade.

On the weekend: Keep it earthy but stylish with tinted moisturizer with SPF, beachy bronzer (applied where the sun would naturally hit the face), a dark brown liner on the top lash line, and tinted lip balm. **Think:** *Elizabeth Olsen*

At work: Try a taupe shimmer eye with mascaraed lashes, peachy cream blush, and a lip that's just a few shades rosier than your natural color.

GLAM GLOBE-TROTTER

At work: Wear luminous taupe/pink/brown eye shadow, a soft glow of pink cream blush, highlighter on the top of your cheekbones, and black mascara. Elegant but easy.

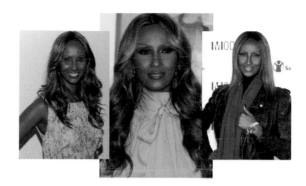

At night: Deepen the eye shadow in the crease and use it as a liner on tops only, or do a thin liquid liner that gets slightly thicker as it works its way outward (iconic chic!). Pair with black volumizing mascara and either a red-stained lip with lip balm top or non-sticky nude gloss.

On the weekend: Trade the shadow for a light beige luminous cream you can apply to your lids for a soft glow. Use a coral blush for a pop of cheek color and wear with nude lipstick or balm and a little mascara. **Think:** *Iman*

MODERN MOVIE STAR

At work: Focus on skin with a sheer luminous foundation, pair with soft pink blush, a stained lip with a gloss in the center, and lots of mascara.

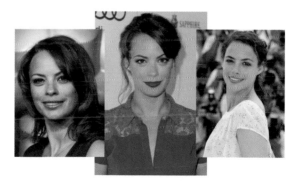

At night: Wing out your black liner or rim your eyes with a gold or gem-toned shadow that picks up a color in your outfit or jewelry, and define your brows. Pair with contoured cheeks and shimmery pink blush on the apples of your cheeks and a red lipstick that's glossy but not too shiny.

On the weekend: The ultimate movie star look—sunscreen. Huge sunglasses. Your favorite lipstick. Chic! **Think:** *Bérénice Bejo*

WORK YOUR
Makeup Budget

IF YOU HAVE $500 TO SPEND ON MAKEUP

Invest in some of my blue-chip lipstick suggestions or create a new makeup kit based on the twenty-one products earlier in this chapter. Or divert some of your budget toward new skin care that will help even out your skin so your makeup looks even better! Save some cash to get your makeup done for your own "red-carpet" event.

IF YOU HAVE $200 TO SPEND

Buy a high-end set of makeup brushes that will last. LA makeup artist Bobby Wells recommends investing in antibacterial synthetic bristles. Use what's left on a new luxurious foundation, NARS the Multiple in Orgasm (you'll feel great every time you use it), and one or two of the blue-chip lipsticks.

IF YOU HAVE $100 TO SPEND

Buy a high-end foundation at a beauty counter or Sephora. Get professional help to try the right shade and maybe wear it today and come back tomorrow and buy it if you really love it. Also pick up a new lipstick and a great cream highlighter or iridescent highlighting moisturizer.

IF YOU HAVE $50 TO SPEND

A new lipstick and shimmer eye shadow stick or two will transform your look.

IF YOU HAVE $20 TO SPEND

Buy a few trendy drugstore items to work with what you already have for the new season: an eye shadow in the color of the moment you can use as both shadow and liner, and a new mascara and false eyelashes to make you feel chic but not broke!

Knowledge: Your Best Makeup Investment

No one purposely wears makeup to make themselves look cheap, but it happens if you don't know any better. I hope this chapter has enlightened you. Remember, it's not money that buys you good taste; it's an open mind, a lot of practice, research, and knowledge that develop your taste. I hope this chapter has given you all that. Whatever you have to spend on your makeup, you're now armed with new makeup wisdom and plenty of affordable products to help you get an upgraded makeup look.

You Don't Have a Dime

- Foundation that doesn't match your skin tone—it's too orange, too dark, too light, too pink, or not blended

- Powder overload—there's no radiance left

- Streaky eighties' style blush

- Bronzer that makes you look orange or muddy

- Harsh eye shadow that's not blended

- Warpaint—dark eye makeup surrounding your eyes actually makes them look tinier

- Clumpy, spiderlike lashes

- Porn-star lip gloss

- Visibly lined lips

- Lipstick on dry, flaky lips

A Million Bucks

- Softened edges, one shade blends into the next

- Foundation you don't even know is there

- Invisible concealer

- Classic makeup with a modern twist

- Makeup that's appropriate for the time and place

- Moist, dewy lips in shades that lift you up

- Glowy cheeks with a beautiful flush

- Eyes that pop in a natural, believable way

- Less-is-more light-handed makeup

- Makeup that gives you confidence and doesn't fixate on your flaws

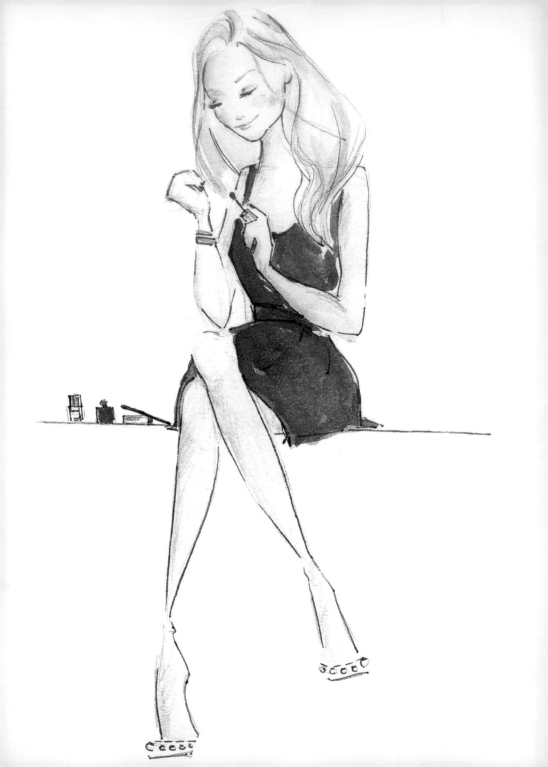

5

From Teeth to Toes and Everywhere in Between

—— The Well-Kept Secrets of Looking Well-Kempt ——

We've talked hair, skin, makeup. Now it's time to move on to the small but important (and sometimes not-so-sexy) things a girl's gotta do to get her glam on. Things like hair removal, dental hygiene, nail care, brow grooming, as well as optional extras like self-tanning. All the details that are easy to forget or neglect but that make a big-bucks difference in how you're perceived. A perfect example of how important good grooming can be? Pippa Middleton. Though she's only related to a future queen, she's a bonafide queen at working the little extra details that make you look well-kempt!

Even though Pippa's bum got all the attention at Kate and Will's wedding, not to mention its own Facebook fan page, you couldn't help but notice her gorgeous bronzed skin (an expensive-looking self-tan, no doubt) or her gorgeous pearly whites. Believe me when I say, neither the tan nor the teeth happened by accident. Because girls like Pippa know that looking expensive is all in the details. They never walk out of the house with chipped polish; they never miss a dentist appointment; they never get caught with hairy legs or brows that need a good plucking. But at the same time, they don't let their beauty life overtake their *real* life.

Women Who Look Too High Maintenance

There's another type of woman we should talk about. This girl is so well-groomed she'd need to be a billionaire (or marry one) to maintain her look. I spent a few summers in Greenwich, Connecticut, sometimes called the Beverly Hills of the East, where I witnessed this breed of over-maintained women firsthand. We're talking tanned legs so smooth they looked like they didn't have a single hair follicle, nails so super-shiny the polish looked as fresh as the *pain au chocolat* in the window of the local bakery, model-perfect brows, and teeth as white as their tennis whites. How did these women pull it off? I heard rumors that one woman in town allegedly spent an entire day each week being pampered inside her stately mansion—massages, facials, mani/pedis, the works. A full day of self-indulgence that didn't buy her happiness (spa treatments can only do so much!) but eventually bought her a divorce. Maybe spending time on her relationship instead of her leg wax would have been a better investment? Ha. I'm just trying to point out that while maintenance is important, you can go overboard. And you can look expensive without going to these kinds of extremes. It all depends on what makes sense for your lifestyle—how much time and money you have and want to put into your look. I know that

Neither the tan nor the teeth happened by accident. Because girls like Pippa know that looking expensive is all in the details.

you have more than manicures to spend time and money on, and so do I. So to get the results you want without becoming a slave to your bikini wax or mani/pedi, my philosophy is: Learn to DIY what you can and leave the rest for the pros. Squeeze those extra beauty services you need into your life, but don't make them your life. Choose salons that get you out of there fast with consistent results and the best prices possible. The goal of good maintenance: To be well-groomed, but not overconsumed—because overdone usually comes off as more trashy than classy. It also makes you look self-absorbed, a trait that's not very pretty.

> *I know that you have more than manicures to spend time and money on, and so do I.*

Brows That Look Low-Brow

Brows frame your face and draw attention to your eyes. At least that's what they're supposed to do. But many women suffer from "low-brow" brow syndrome, brows that draw attention to themselves instead of to you, symptoms of which include unflattering shape and color, phony fill-in, and a general lack of attention. Because your eyes are the first things people notice about you, your brows are always in the spotlight. Luckily, changing your brows isn't that hard to do.

Find Your Best Brow Shape

A brow makeover, like a manicure, can instantly upgrade your look. I always suggest letting your brows grow out, having them professionally shaped, and then keeping up with the maintenance yourself. If you use a magnifying mirror and pluck only the hairs that are growing in, you can get by with one professional appointment per season, or even less. But whether you go pro or DIY, it's important to know how to find your best shape. The most fail-safe solution? "Always stay as close to the natural shape as possible, which usually follows the line of your brow bone," says brow artist Luba Tadova, of New York's Laura Geller Makeup Studio, the only one who ever touches my brows besides me. Here's some more advice from Luba to help you get your own personal best shape.

- **Customize your brows to your features.** Smaller eyes look better with fuller brows; bigger eyes can go thinner.

- **Brows should help define the contours of your face.** Go for a more arched shape if your face is round or full; flatter, narrower brows if your face is long or narrow.

- **To create the best arch,** be sure to pluck right under the highest point of your natural arch and then work the rest to balance the line of the whole brow.

- **Brows should start above the corner of your eye,** but keep a natural edge; pluck away only hairs you need to between your brows (if you have a unibrow, waxing is best). An exception to this is if you have deep-set eyes, for which tweezing a little on each side at the start of your brows can make you look more wide-eyed.

- **Shaping the top of brows is tricky and not necessary.** A pro may sometimes do it to enhance your shape, but don't touch the top yourself.

- **When shaping at home,** Luba suggests drawing the shape and width you want right on your brows with a white pencil and then plucking the ones that fall out of place.

CREATE YOUR OWN BROW BOARD

Celebrity brows can provide great inspiration, or help you learn what you like if you DIY or "talk the talk" for better communication with a brow pro. Tear out photos from magazines or get to work on Google to find out brows you love, then pin them all up on a board or paste them into a folder —you may notice trends that appeal to you in terms of arch shape, width, and whether the brows go up or down at the ends. You can then take the photos with you when you get your brows done.

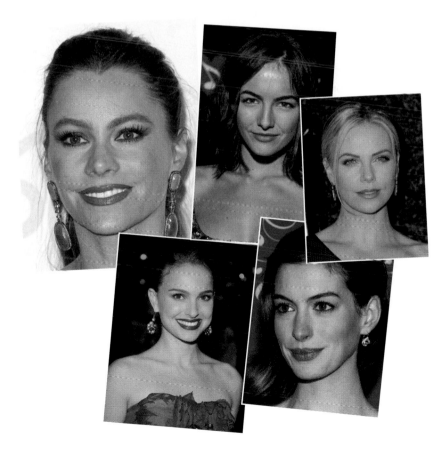

The Top Eight Brow Mistakes

According to Brett Freedman—the celebrity brow whiz I introduced you to in the makeup chapter, who tends (or should I say mends!) the brows of hundreds of women a year, including stars like Catherine Zeta-Jones— these are the biggest brow shape mistakes women make, along with solutions, whether you fix them yourself or invest in a single professional brow shape you can upkeep afterward. In most cases, you'll have to let your brows grow back first to have something to work with.

THE MISTAKE

The Obvious Fill-in Brow

These are brows filled in or elongated with the wrong-colored powder or pencil, or brows that look like makeup, not hair. Most women go too dark, which makes the brows look heavy, artificial, and blocklike, or use straight strokes that look like they're drawn on.

THE FIX

Use a powder or pencil at least a few shades lighter than the color of your hair and apply in small strokes to mimic hair and give a 3-D effect.

If you're blonde to medium brown, a taupe pencil (sometimes called beige) is best (if you've got golden highlights in your hair, go with a golden taupe as opposed to an ashy taupe).

If you're dark brunette, go for a lighter brown; **raven-haired,** a dark brown.

If you're a super-pale blonde with matching, almost invisible brows (whether they're natural or bleached-out along with your hair), you need to go slightly darker to define your brows, but not so dark that they look artificial.

If you're a redhead, choose a soft auburn.

If you're still not sure what shade to choose, taupe is a fail-safe—it'll give your brows enough of a shadow to look less sparse without being obvious.

THE MISTAKE

The "Block" Brow

Brows that look too hard-edged and structured, no femininity

THE FIX

Skip the fill-in entirely if you don't already and take yourself to a pro without passing go. You're the lucky one with enough hair there to get a new look pronto. Ask for a nice arched effect.

THE MISTAKE

The "Anorexic" Brow

Brows that are too thin to do their job—which is to frame your face and accent your eyes—or so painfully thin they look obviously over-plucked

THE FIX

Fill them in lightly and slightly while you let them grow; but often brows that have been plucked again and again never do grow out. Beverly Hills celebrity dermatologist Boris Zaks tells me using Latisse grows brows, too, though it's not approved by the FDA for this purpose. Ask your dermatologist.

THE MISTAKE

The Droopy Brow

Brows that go down at the end, drawing the eyes down instead of lifting them up. Important to consider as you get older, when the skin around your eyes is starting to droop—why play it up?

THE FIX

You may be able to just tweeze off a few stray hairs at the end of your brows to straighten them out, but you may also want to try letting your brows grow out completely before having them reshaped at an upward slant. It'll act like an eye lift!

THE MISTAKE

The "Sperm/Tadpole Look"

Brows that look like a ball with a tail coming out of it—they're missing the middle!

THE FIX

You're going to have to let the area between the ball and tail grow back and have it shaped into a more gradual transition. But in the meantime, fill in from the area between the ball and the peak of the arch, adding back the missing triangle shape to blend in the two parts of your brow, creating a more gradual arch.

THE MISTAKE

The "Surprised" Look

Round brows that are semicircles with no arch. They make a woman look like she's constantly in a state of surprise.

THE FIX

While they grow out, tweeze only the "homeless" strays that are way below your brows or edging toward your temples. Use a brow powder to fill in sparse areas as brows grow back (and if they don't, follow the advice for anorexic brows on the previous page). To reshape them, the pro will re-create an arch for you and lift the ends up instead of down.

THE MISTAKE

The Contrived "Over-Arch"

Brows with an overdone arch so high it looks artificial. Or they arch in the wrong place.

THE FIX

Use a brow pencil or powder on both sides of the arch to lower it a bit and make it look less severe while brows grow in. Then have a pro create a more natural-looking arch over your iris.

THE MISTAKE

Messy Brows

Brows with stray hairs growing out from the last tweeze beneath your brow line, or hairs you forgot to tweeze in the first place. "Not removing the homeless hairs that grow sparsely from the tail to the temple is one of the most common brow mistakes," says Freedman.

THE FIX

Clean them up! Just tweezing strays to clean up your brows without even changing the shape makes a big difference. To get those hard-to-grab growing-in hairs (the ones that look like little black dots . . . hate them!), pull out that magnifying mirror. And here's a weird idea—pluck in a car parked outside. The overhead mirror is the right height and angle, you can adjust your seat to get close to it, and the daylight helps illuminate strays.

That Million-Dollar Smile!

Expensive teeth are hard to miss. They're radiant, polished, bright, and white (but not so white they look fake!). They glow. They shine. They're the smile that lights up your face . . . and the whole room. Tacky teeth on the other hand are chipped, dull, stained, and obviously not very well-maintained. Most of us sit somewhere in the middle of these two extremes. "Actresses, models, and celebrities take serious care of their smile, they know it can be a real asset," says one of the founders of modern cosmetic dentistry, celebrity dentist Irwin Smigel. And there are plenty of civilian women who fall into this category, too—they're the ones you see flossing or brushing their teeth in the office bathroom. On the other hand are those of us who brush twice a day, maybe floss, but that's about it. You can get away with this, but it won't give you a million-dollar smile. So let's talk about what will.

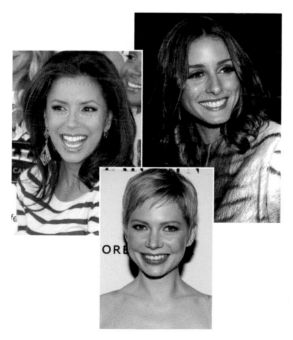

A PIECE OF SMILE ADVICE EVEN MONEY CAN'T BUY

There's one smile you can't buy (because it's not for sale): a smile that comes from self-assurance, inner happiness, and self-confidence, not the dentist's office. Sure, whiter, brighter teeth or dental enhancements (veneers and the like) can help give you that confidence, but it's very possible all you need to have a million-dollar smile is a toothbrush, some Crest Whitestrips, and a new attitude. In other words, to make over your smile, you may just have to use it more.

The Souped-up Smile Maintenance Plan

Brush Longer

Dr. Smigel tells his patients to spend a whole two minutes brushing their teeth to thoroughly remove plaque, followed by flossing once a day. Sounds time-consuming but it's just five minutes total.

Add a Mouth Rinse to Your Regime

Choose one without alcohol, which can dry out tooth enamel, leaving it susceptible to staining. Especially effective are mouth rinses that contain antioxidants. PerioSciences AO ProRinse is a good example.

The Right Toothpaste

The simplest brightening strategy is to use a nonabrasive whitening toothpaste. Choose one with ingredients less likely to cause tooth sensitivity, like Calprox (Supersmile), carbamide peroxide, or urea peroxide (Rembrandt). Or go for a green brightener that removes stains via kaolin, a nonabrasive natural clay (Dentisse) or baking soda (Arm & Hammer toothpastes). Important note: "They don't work on veneers or other dental work, and you should never use them more than directed," stresses another top New York dentist, Dr. Sheldon Nadler.

Add Extra Whitening Oomph!

Try Crest Whitestrips, which will give you whiter teeth in two to four weeks. A whitening accelerator used before your whitening toothpaste, like Supersmile Professional Activating Rods or Arm & Hammer Whitening Booster 3X, can give a similar effect, preparing your teeth's surface for the whitening ingredient in the toothpaste. Make sure to take the recommended break between cycles so as not to damage enamel or sensitize teeth.

Smile Makeovers at the Dentist's Office

- **The most cost-efficient way to significantly improve your smile:** Professional whitening, which can reverse many years of stain buildup for $250–$1,000—a lot less than other in-office smile makeover methods. Dr. Nadler prefers the tray method over lasers for its longer-lasting, least-sensitizing results—your dentist makes you custom-fitted trays you wear at home for thirty minutes a day using a special whitening solution.

- **Next up on the bang for your buck scale:** Bonding with composite resin, a noninvasive procedure to mask imperfections and change the shape of teeth without the high price of the crown jewel of dentistry—porcelain veneers.

- **The high-priced big hitter:** Porcelain veneers, ceramic covers that can reshape teeth to create more attractive shapes while covering up things that cheapen a smile like chipping, odd shapes, spaces between teeth, dull surfaces, and yellowing. The cost of such a procedure can be in the thousands, expensive but worth it if you hate your smile and can afford it.

- **For the most natural look:** Whether you're whitening your own teeth or having them covered with porcelain or resin, the trick to keeping them looking real (and not reality star) is to never go whiter than the whites of your eyes.

Celebrity Smile Secrets

- **Drink a glass of water after you eat** to wash off anything that might stain, but especially after soy sauce and ketchup, coffee, tea, and alcohol (even white wine—the acidity can stain over time).

- **Wet your teeth with your tongue before a picture**—it creates a luster.

- **Wear a blue-based red lipstick**—it'll make your teeth look whiter and brighter.

- **Sparkly earrings** can also reflect brightness on your teeth, but avoid gold because it tends to exaggerate yellow tones.

- **Snack on apples and celery** between meals—they have a natural abrasiveness to scrub off food particles. Strawberries have natural bleaching properties.

- **Brush your teeth before going out.** It removes a natural film that lives on your teeth, making it less likely that food or drinks will stick to them.

- **Stop smoking.** 'Nuf said.

- **Use on-the-go teeth and breath fresheners,** like Colgate Wisp and Supersmile Quikees and Professional Whitening Gum.

Nails: The Ultimate Cheap Thrill

Moving right down your body, let's touch on nails. They may be small but they make a big impact. A bottle of the latest straight-off-the-runway Chanel polish won't break your bank but it will make you feel incredibly chic and expensive. There are so many great color and texture options out there, nail polish is now like "fast fashion," easy and inexpensive to buy to add a little newness to your look, to try on color trends, or to accessorize yourself for the new season. The easiest, most affordable part of you to makeover—a little TLC and presto-polish-chango is all it takes to turn nasty "before" nails into flauntable "afters."

I actually find when my nails are a mess, I feel like a mess. You might call it beauty therapy—as soon as I get my nails done, I'm back in control again. Polished nails equal polished life! No wonder *The New York Times* calls nail polish the new lipstick indicator, referring to the economic theory that women spend money on small indulgences—traditionally lipsticks, more recently nail polishes—when the economy dips!

When beautifully maintained, nails are another piece of the puzzle that makes you look well-groomed; when neglected or ignored, they make you look unkempt, even if the rest of you is very well-kempt. If you're looking at your hands now and cringing, no guilt—nail care slip-ups happen to the best of us. As Beverly Hills nail pro Kimmie Kyees says, "A cheap nail maybe once was a nice manicure that's just been on too long."

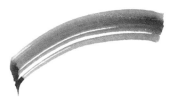

NAIL MISHAPS

Cheap-looking nails fall into two categories: nail neglect and bad taste. And it isn't difficult to fix mistakes in either of these categories. It's just a matter of knowing better and caring enough to put in the effort. These nail mistakes are easily cured by high-tailing it to a manicurist or scheduling your own DIY digit downtime:

Lack-of-Attention Nail Mistakes

Chipped polish

Jagged edges

Mixed lengths

Raggedy cuticles

Long toenails

Cracked heels

Bad Taste Mistakes

Nails that are past a natural-looking length

Long, square nails—the fakest looking nails you can have

Phony-looking acrylics

Airbrushed nails—these can look cool on a trendy person, but they don't look expensive.

Neons—hard to pull off

What Makes a Nail Look Expensive?

Three Rather Simple Things

The Shape

Two chic shapes to try:

The almond—Fashion-savvy New York and Hollywood manicurists tell me there's been a new direction on the runway and
with celebrities to go a little longer—definitely not too long,
unless you're Rihanna—but long enough to make an oval. "It's
a medium-length nail that says 'What dishes? I treat my nails
like jewels, and I take care of them like I do my other luxury
accessories,' says manicurist Roxanne Valinoti of Creative Nail
Design (CND).

A squoval (square + oval) is a go-to shape you can't go wrong
with. Essentially a rounded top with squared edges, it's pretty
break-proof and easy to file (making it a great shape to ask for
at an $8 manicure). A chic tweak is the "Jin Soon" shape named
by and for eponymous manicurist Jin Soon Choi. Just the opposite of a squoval, it's flat on top with rounded edges. Quick side
story: I helped Jin get her first agent years ago, and now she's the
backstage nail guru at shows like Oscar de la Renta with A-list
movie stars clawing for her manicures.

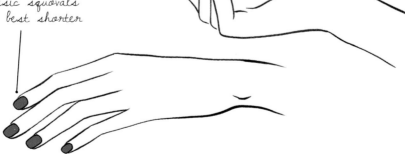

almonds are a new, longer shape

classic squovals look best shorter

Attention to Detail

This means nails that look like you care about them. All of the tips below you can DIY, and you should expect them at a quality salon.

- **Take the time to file your nails** if they grow out or need some lovin' before your next manicure.

- **Use a cuticle oil every day** to prevent cuticles from drying out.

- **Trim stray cuticles** instead of ignoring them.

- **Moisturize your hands** and take care of the skin that surrounds the nail, not just the nail itself, a place inexpensive manicure places often skimp.

- **Make sure the polish fits the frame of your nail,** not wandering over the border onto your skin. Apply polish in thin coats for a smooth finish.

- **Be sure to seal the sides** or the edge of the tip of your nail with polish.

- **If one nail breaks, then file them all** to a uniform length.

The Color

You might be surprised to hear that almost any color—except neons—can look expensive today, as long as the polish is well-applied, has a high shine (splurge on a quality topcoat), works with your skin tone (don't just wear a trendy color if it doesn't look good on you), and is applied to well-maintained hands. But the shades to follow are chicest:

Nail Colors That Make You Look Expensive

THE NUDES

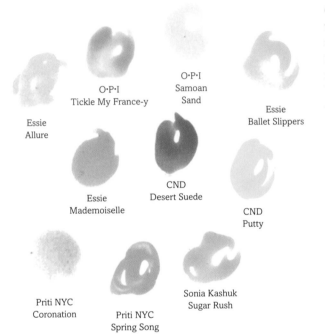

Essie
Allure

O·P·I
Tickle My France-y

O·P·I
Samoan
Sand

Essie
Ballet Slippers

Essie
Mademoiselle

CND
Desert Suede

CND
Putty

Priti NYC
Coronation

Priti NYC
Spring Song

Sonia Kashuk
Sugar Rush

Classic sheer pink— the ultimate in low maintenance—always looks clean and chic. Sure, it's been around the block but sometimes it's just what you need. Personally, I like a beigier nude for a more natural effect. You can update a sheer nude manicure with a sparkle, pearl, or shimmer topcoat.

Skin-tone nudes are a bit more opaque and they're a chic new option—low maintenance, high style—that elongates your fingers and makes your legs look longer when you wear them on your toes.

TAUPES AND GRAYS

Unconventional colors started as a trend but are now a chic and fashionable, go-with-everything classic. Choose a deep tone for the richest look.

CND
Chocolate Milk

Essie
Chinchilly

O·P·I
You Don't Know Jacques!

REDS

Classic red is a no-brainer—chic, sexy, Marilyn Monroe (or Scarlett Johansson)–esque.

Blue-based red is easier to wear and chicer than tomato-y orange reds.

Deep reds and burgundies look more modern and fashion-forward than bright reds but have become just as classic.

CND
Dark Ruby

CND
Rouge Red

Essie
Fifth Avenue

Essie
Wicked

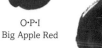

O·P·I
Big Apple Red

Priti NYC
Queen of the
Night Tulip

Deborah Lippmann
My Old Flame

O·P·I
Malaga Wine

DEEP, DARK JEWEL TONES

Priti NYC
Magic Man Iris

O·P·I
Russian Navy

Essie
Bobbing for Baubles

Gem-tone polishes like emerald greens, amethyst purples, and icy deep sapphire blues, bedazzle your hands almost like the real thing! If they feel too trendy on your fingers, they'll look gorgeous on your toes.

O·P·I
Lincoln Park After Dark

CND
Inkwell

A Celebrity Nail Pro's Tricks to Prettier Feet

Roxanne Valinoti of CND is my backstage go-to nail expert during Fashion Week. She sees twenty to thirty models per show, times twenty shows per season, so she knows models don't have the prettiest feet—all that walking and ill-fitting shoes. Her great tricks can help your feet look better even without a pedicure:

- **Shoes, please.** Don't walk around barefoot—it wreaks havoc on your feet.

- **Save your flip-flops for the beach.** "They're so bad for your feet, especially if you live in a city. Your feet will become black and your heels will crack."

- **Exfoliate your feet in the shower.** Roxanne uses a regular nail file instead of a pumice stone, which she says are terrible for feet. She prefers to start with a coarse grit foot file and then finish with a fine grit file.

- **Give your feet a softening hot-oil treatment.** Warm up olive oil for ten seconds in the microwave, then soak your feet for ten minutes (being sure to wipe them afterward so you don't slip!).

- **To lighten yellow-stained toenails,** drop a denture cream tablet into a bowl of water and dip your feet into it for about 5 minutes—it's safer than bleach or peroxide . . . "And it works!" says Roxanne. Afterward, do a light buff and then massage feet with moisturizer. If you do this before bed, sleep in socks.

THE INSTANT GRATIFICATION EMERGENCY MANICURE

What to do when you don't have time for a manicure and your nails are a mess?

If you have 30 seconds

Take off the polish and moisturize your hands. It's better to go bare and have nothing on than to wear old polish.

If you have 2 minutes

Take off the polish, quickly file nails, and push your cuticles back with a wet towel. Check for hangnails and nip if needed. Apply a sheer polish or, even faster, buff your nails to high shine.

Try Revlon Crazy Shine, $3.49; or CND Girlfriend Buffer, $7.95.

How to Get an Expensive Manicure at a Cheap Nail Salon

Don't get me wrong—there's talent everywhere—but in case you don't find it, here's how to get a spa-finish result at the local nail bar.

- **Ask for a rounded square.** Not all manicurists are familiar with the squoval term.

- **Make all nails the same length.** A good idea at any manicure but especially important at a walk-in salon. It's important to maintain the same length with all ten fingers, even if it means chopping nine to match one shorter one, because if you don't, it looks like you need to file your nails.

- **Stick to the basics.** Skip gels, enhancements, acrylics, or fake nails. I've had Shellac done on the cheap but it peeled right off.

- **Find a salon with a sense of fashion and style,** even if it's not high-end. Check CND and O·P·I website locators for salons they've actually trained (as opposed to ones who just buy the product).

- **Call ahead for an appointment.** Even if you don't need one. By scheduling the time for you, they'll probably spend more time on you.

- **Alternatively, get just a polish change at an expensive salon**—a high-quality finish often at half the price of a full high-end manicure.

THE GEL NAIL CRAZE: SHOULD YOU BUY IN?

A manicure that looks freshly polished for two weeks sounds like a dream, and if you can't get your butt to the manicurist enough or want to wear color without it chipping in a day, the service is a godsend . . . if you can afford it. You'll pay on average twice the price of a regular manicure. But it's really not that bad if you think of it like prepaying for coffee with a Starbucks card—you know you'll spend it eventually anyway. I'd avoid the old gel services that require soaking them off in acetone and stick to the name services like Shellac from CND and O·P·I's Colorgel, which have less damaging wrap-removal systems. The former is cured with UV light, the latter with LED light. I do find my nails need a break after multiple gel manicures in a row, so I save them for before vacations or busy weeks.

BOOK AN APPOINTMENT WITH...

KIMMIE KYEES
The Polish Perfectionist

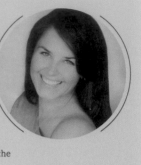

As a mobile manicurist, Kimmie's celebrity roster includes the likes of Jennifer Lopez, Rihanna, Kate Bosworth, and Katy Perry. Her celeb list is so long it means more to say who she hasn't done than who she has! Kimmie travels with about three hundred colors so she has anything a celebrity, director, or editor wants. In the off chance she doesn't have the perfect color in her collection, she'll custom-blend it.

KIMMIE KYEES'S LITTLE BLACK BAG

Here's what's in the tool kit Kimmie schleps to her Hollywood house calls:

The little extra something: River stones

The soak: SpaRitual Harmonizing Soak Tonic

The cuticle pusher-backer: Bellissima

The cuticle nipper: O·P·I AccuNip

The exfoliator: Orly SugarFIX

The massage cream: SpaRitual Organic Moisturizer

The pre-base coat: Orly Bonder Rubberized Polish Gripping Basecoat

The polish: O·P·I, NARS, M·A·C, and Ginger + Liz, a fashion-forward vegan line

The top coat: Seche Vite

The Shine Formula: Orly Flash Dry Quick-Dry Shine Drops and CND SolarSpeed Spray (the combo smells so good, she calls it the "dessert" of her manicure!)

Kimmie's Pet Peeve

"Pay attention to the cuticles; you can have a perfect paint job and no hangnails, but if you have dry, crunchy cuticles it just looks undone," she says.

Kimmie's Cheap Trick

Dry nail polish from the drugstore, like Sally Hansen Salon Effects Real Nail Polish Strips—adhesive polish stickers.

AT-HOME CELEBRITY MANI/PEDI

by Kimmie Kyees

The difference between a professional and home mani/pedi is the little extras. They don't take long, and they make you feel pampered, your skin softer, and your polish longer lasting. Kimmie Kyees fills us in!

1. TAKE OFF THE OLD COLOR and apply cuticle remover.

2. SOAK HANDS in a bowl of warm water, but add something special like flower petals, aromatherapy oil, or Kimmie's signature—river stones you can pick up at a nursery—as well as a moisturizing bath soak.

3. PUSH BACK THE CUTICLES with a cuticle stick or tool, nip away excess cuticles and file one hand into the desired shape, always filing in one direction with hands open instead of in a fist. Soak that hand and repeat on the other hand.

4. EXFOLIATE HANDS OR FEET up to your elbows or knees with a gentle abrasive scrub.

5. MASSAGE TIME. Using a thick moisturizer massage up to your elbow or knee, five minutes each hand/foot.

6. WIPE EACH NAIL with polish remover to rid any lotion or oil that'll prevent polish adhesion. Then apply a basecoat that balances nail pH to help polish adhere.

7. APPLY two coats of polish and a topcoat, allowing each coat to dry before starting the next one. The trick, she says, is to cover the nail all the way from left to right, being sure to start right at the cuticle, then cap the end with the color and top coat so it won't chip as quickly.

8. IMMEDIATELY use a clean-up brush (an old polish brush or even an eyeliner brush will work) to clean up the edges and remove excess polish, both clear and colored.

9. HER SECRET SHINE FORMULA: Wait two minutes after applying the topcoat, then apply fast-dry drops. Wait another two minutes and spritz hands with a fast-dry spray—it makes the skin look well-moisturized, and the polish dries fast and lasts longer.

DIY POLISH LIKE A PRO

Buy professional nail polishes.
Priced between drugstore and prestige, they give you
the high-shine, high-quality look of a pro manicure. Try brands
like CND, O•P•I, Priti NYC, Essie, and Deborah Lippmann.

At the drugstore, skip fast-drying polishes.
They tend to dull; consider a pro topcoat for a high-shine finish,
even if you wear drugstore polish.

To apply polish to your nondominant hand:
Steady it on a table first. Polishing in mid-air doesn't work.

Clean up the edges with a Q-tip dipped in polish remover.
Wait until your nails are dry so you can hold the Q-tip with a
steadier hand without taking off your polish!

Sandwich your color between a basecoat and topcoat.
This makes it stick, seals it on, and adds shine.

Don't try to fix a smudge.
Start over.

You can't save chipped color.
Take it off and start over. If you apply another coat on top
you'll see the old color around the edges—can you say cheesy?

Couturize Your Nails

PARK AVENUE PRETTY

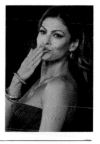

Manicure: Either nude and natural—maybe a sheer pink with a gold or pearlized overlay—or choose from my Nail Colors That Make You Look Expensive Swatches on page 166–167.

Pedicure: Anything goes! Try a color you love but wouldn't wear on your fingers because it's not classic enough for you.

HOLLYWOOD BOHO

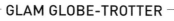

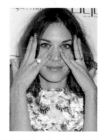

Manicure: Go for dark neutrals—grays and browns.

Pedicure: Try an offbeat shade with an iridescent finish or go for deep, dark jewel tones—emeralds, deep icy blue, deep and/or shimmery purple.

GLAM GLOBE-TROTTER

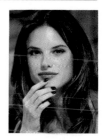

Manicure: A brush-on gel manicure to give your nails a great-looking, long-lasting (two weeks) look you won't have to think about. Try a chic taupe, vampy red, chic purple, or deep almost black nail.

Pedicure: Go dark and sexy with a matte finish or keep it neutral with flesh-toned opaque nail polish.

MODERN MOVIE STAR

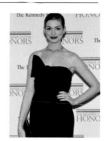

Manicure: Go bright and sexy with the latest takes on reds (always classic and classy), or try a flesh-tone nude with a special effects shimmer—it'll make your hands look long and feminine.

Pedicure: Opaque polish that matches your skintone to elongate your legs in stilettos (they become one long line), or match your toenails to your sandals or your dress (bring a swatch to the nail salon).

Hair Removal: Smooth Moves to Fit Your Body and Budget

Now it's time for the not-so-sexy and sometimes painful maintenance stuff—hair removal. Another nitty-gritty detail you need to sweat to look well-groomed! Whether you go low-cost razor, high-end laser, or not-as-taxing waxing, there are plenty of options to get you sleek and smooth. One way to save on professional hair-removal services is to decide where on your body you really need it. For most women, the bikini area is the best investment—it's hard to get great DIY results down there! After that, analyze your time and budget to see if you want to add legs or arms to the equation—tops, bottoms, or both? Let's look at some options to help you get smooth and sleek whatever your price range.

> *Never skimp on quality, even if you like the price.*

Lasers: High-Maintenance Splurge, No-Maintenance Results

Very rich girls—the super high-maintenance kind I mentioned who look like they don't have any hair follicles? They've lasered away every last hair from their bikini line to their arms and legs, even their armpits. That sounds extreme, but lately laser hair removal isn't just for millionairesses! More and more women are looking at laser hair removal as a good investment, with its ability to outright banish ingrowns and make monthly waxing visits and oh-my-god-I-forgot-to-shave emergencies obsolete. If you can make the upfront investment in both time and money, you're left with not just low-maintenance legs, but no-maintenance legs. Sure, it's a lot faster and cheaper to shave—lasering requires a series of appointments every four to six weeks for a period of time—and can cost you thousands per body part. But when you add up the price of monthly waxing appointments, and compare that figure to the cost of lasering, plenty of women feel justified in the expenditure and say it may actually be cheaper in the long run. To cut costs, consider just doing one part of your body—most women start with their bikini line.

Here are some tips for getting good-quality laser results at the best price possible:

- **Never skimp on quality, even if you like the price.** Lasers work by killing the hair at the follicle with extreme heat—and if not done properly you could get burned or scarred. If you have any creepy feelings when you walk into the reception area or even when you're lying on the table, hightail it out of there!

- **Determine whether laser will work on your skin tone.** Not all lasers work on darker or tanned skin because they have trouble detecting the hair. It's not a bad idea to go to a laser specialist who works within a doctor's office to be sure you're a good candidate for it in the first place.

- **Do your research.** Laser technology is changing all the time, too, so it pays to be informed about your options before you plunk down cash on a laser system that's out of date. New lasers like the Soprano XLi can not only treat more skin tones but also they hurt less!

- **Save without sacrificing quality.** Look for specials on websites like Groupon and Lifebooker. Even the most high-end spas will offer better prices online or during slow times to boost business.

HAIR REMOVAL WITHOUT THE PAIN

- **Make sure you time it right!** "Your endorphins are naturally higher in the morning so an A.M. appointment is the best. Also, waxing will hurt more during your period so try to time it a week or two away," says Katherine Goldman, the owner of LA celebrity waxing hot spot Stript Wax Bar.

- **Take a pain reliever like Motrin** an hour before your appointment to help with the pain as well. After hair removal, apply cortisone and aloe to alleviate redness and swelling.

- **Ask your dermatologist for a prescription numbing cream,** like Emla or lidocaine. The catch is you have to remember to apply it half an hour before the appointment. It won't take the pain away but it will take the edge off.

- **Avoid alcohol and coffee** before a session to make the process more comfortable.

- **Be consistent in your visits.** If done once a month, waxing barely hurts because the hair is sparse and not too long. If you take off months during the winter or whenever, it'll grow back and be as bad as the first time. Plus once you ignore it, it's easy to keep ignoring it.

- **If you do get an ingrown hair, don't pick.** A little Neosporin, acne medication, or tea tree oil can help clear it. Using a salicylic or alpha hydroxy acid facial pad down there will help open the pores and prevent ingrowns.

Not-So-Taxing Waxing: Great Results for Less Money and Pain!

I'm still a wax girl, in spite of the convenience and permanence of laser hair removal. And, luckily, waxing is becoming easier and more affordable than ever. I don't know if you've noticed but waxing salons or spas—places that specialize in waxing and offer no other services—are popping up in more cities across the country. Though it's not like manicures where you can find a salon on every corner, there may be a franchised waxing studio near you that'll offer the services you want at a price you can afford. I go to the Uni K Wax Center chain and find they're geniuses at giving you excellent, consistent results at a great price. My bikini wax—including the front (is that TMI? Probably.)—costs just $25 and is so pain-free I almost feel like I'm at a spa. They use a green proprietary natural wax that contains pine sap, beeswax, and aloe vera, and each client gets their very own freshly sterilized container that is emptied afterward (no worries about double-dipping!). It's done without strips and the waxers get intensive training, making for a speedy, efficient, consistently good service. Though not all waxing salons/bars are as consistent, Uni K has figured it out. I'm not the only one hooked on their waxing. Beyoncé, Ashanti, America Ferrera, and Cameron Diaz—all of whom can afford to spend more than $25 on their bikini wax—go there, too. I also like that you can book online and can make an appointment any time of the day or night—during a workday I'm not usually thinking about waxing and that's how those hair-removal emergencies happen!

Your Bikini Area

Waxing wins hands down in my book as the best option for your bikini line. You need to first decide on the look you want—a regular bikini wax where they just clean up the sides? A Brazilian bikini wax where they take it all off unless you instruct them otherwise? (Be sure to ask what they consider a Brazilian, by the way, so there are no surprises.) Do you want a strip left in front, and if so, straight and narrow or more triangular like a martini glass? Do you want to take hair off the top as well as the sides?

For a less expensive bill at the end, be sure to ask specifically what the service you choose includes (or read up on it on the spa menu if you're too embarrassed to ask). If you like a little more hair removed here or there it's often cheaper to ask for it on the waxing table rather than booking it outright—you can up your tip if she doesn't add it to the bill.

Legs

Tops, bottoms, or both? Skipping the full leg in favor of just the thighs is a huge money-saver if you laser or wax. You can shave the bottoms as lots of impatient women like me do—who wants to sport the hairy leg look while you wait for it to grow in anyway?

Arms

I'm not big on arm waxing—I think some hair there looks more natural—but if your hair is really dark or heavy, it's your best choice. Decide if you can get away with just the forearms or if you want to go for your upper arms too. Bleaching is another option, but best if your hair is dark but not too heavy or full (in which case it'll be just as noticeable when you bleach it, maybe more so depending on your skin tone). See a pro for best results or use an at-home kit, being sure to remove the formula a few minutes early so you don't overbleach.

Facial Hair

Waxing wins for mustache, light peach fuzz, and nose hair, but for heavier or darker peach fuzz and/or those annoying chin hairs (why are they always black????), you might consider a more permanent hair-removal option. Besides lasers (be sure to see a pro! It's your face!), there's electrolysis, but I find that procedure painful, tedious, and slow—a little like seeing a shrink who never graduates you. I'm more into instant gratification if you haven't noticed! Bleaching works, too, but remember it can backfire—platinum hair stands out just as much as dark hair on dark skin tones.

Taking It All Off at Home

Shaving

For ease and affordability, you can't beat shaving. And I know you know how to do it, so I won't go there except to recommend that you get yourself a really good razor that contours to your body and has built-in lubrication. I use the Schick Intuition. It has the lubrication inside it, allowing for fast, flawless results. It's genius. If you must shave dry without a lubricated razor, use a body oil to help the razor slide.

Nair

Hair-removal experts are mixed on products like Nair. Some say they promote ingrowns because only the hair on top is washed away, leaving the hair beneath the skin on it's own to break through. Others question the chemicals they contain. I'm not going to recommend these as your regular hair removal method for all of the above possible negatives, although they do seem more foolproof than at-home waxing kits, which can hurt.

Waxing

With waxing getting so inexpensive, I'd prefer that you don't try to do it yourself, but if you want to, choose cold waxing strips you apply without heat—they're much less of a mess.

LIDIA TIVICHI'S DIY WAX RULES

1. Make sure the skin has no oil or cream on it before you wax.

2. Apply baby powder to the area to sop up sweat that would interfere with the wax.

3. Apply the wax strip with enough pressure that you'll be able to yank it off.

4. Pull skin in one direction with one hand to make it tight, then quickly pull off the strip with the other hand.

BOOK AN APPOINTMENT WITH...

LIDIA TIVICHI
The Waxer with a Wait List

When Lidia Tivichi tells you she'll squeeze you in when she opens at 6 A.M., you make sure you're there at 5:59. This Romanian blonde dynamo has a clientele that runs the gamut from top magazine editors to celebrities like Gwyneth Paltrow (who told Lidia she wants to clone her!) to the Upper East Side types you'd see on *Gossip Girl* . . . with plenty of Manhattan moms and regular everyday girls thrown in to the mix. After her warp-speed waxing, she'll apply a soothing customized concoction of aloe vera gel, zinc oxide, and camphor, all from the drugstore, leaving it on to be washed off at home if the client's skin is red and irritated.

"One place it's okay to be tacky: Your bikini wax! If you want to go heart-shaped, bedazzled, or va-tooed (preferably temporary), I won't scold you. No one sees it so it's a perfect place to bring out your inner trashiness!"

—Lidia Tivichi

Lidia's Pet Peeve
"Body hair at the beach. I see so many hairy people in bathing suits, I want to bring my table to the beach and wax them for free!"

Lidia's Favorite Cheap Tricks
Bacitracin, Aquaphor, or Neosporin used for three days after waxing to prevent ingrowns.

An alpha hydroxy acid rinse or skin care product every day afterward to help keep pores open, so hair can break through without becoming irritated.

Self-Tanning: Your Best Friend or Worst Enemy

Self-tanning may not even be on your maintenance radar, but for women in the public eye—celebs, royalty, fashion designers, models, et cetera—it's kind of like getting a manicure: a must, not a maybe! In fact, it's got a new name: skin finishing! Women who regularly slip into revealing gowns for the red carpet or for formal events consider the look of their body skin just as important as the skin on their face, and the tan is kind of like semipermanent makeup, ensuring a good "foundation" for whatever they put on top, almost like an invisible body shaper. Why all the fuss? Besides being obviously safer than the real thing, a self-tan can make you look healthier, well rested, sexier, like you just got back from St. Barts or live an otherwise chichi life. It can hide things like cellulite and visible veins and mosquito bite scars, even shape and contour your body, making you look more toned and fit. It can even give you the cheekbones of a supermodel without a trip to a plastic surgeon. And along with doing all this it can boost your confidence, big-time, so that you feel better, dressed or undressed. That's the upside. On the downside: A self-tan that looks orange, streaky, or obviously not real is totally tacky. So how to get the good tan, the one that looks natural and golden, not garish?

Four Secrets to an Expensive Self-Tan

1 **An expensive tan is a couture tan,** meaning it's customized to each wearer. Some high-end salons, like Chocolate Sun in LA, actually hand-mix custom formulas; others use one standard formula that adjusts to each wearers' natural skin tone, applying it in layers to customize the color on the body. One way to customize your own tan is to use both a body tanner and a face tanner, as well as a diluted body tanner on the places that would get less natural sun (see The Custom-Blended Tan on page 182).

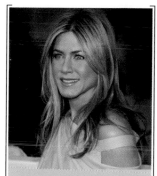

Jennifer Aniston's
faux-real bronze glow

2 **An expensive tan slims and contours your body.** A celebrity tan isn't just painted on as if it were house paint. Top tanning artists use their medium to create the illusion of thinner thighs, tighter abs, and more-toned triceps. Almost like temporary plastic surgery, they can even create the effect of higher cheekbones! Face contouring can be done at home; you can get similar body-contouring done at a spray-tan salon—just ask for it.

3 **An expensive tan takes work, time, and money.** Women who wear these beautiful tans, like Jennifer Aniston, usually have to have a serious maintenance regime to prevent them from getting dark and dirty-looking or patchy, all of which make a tan look tacky. That involves at-home or professional exfoliation to get rid of the old tan before the new one goes on and reapplications at least twice a week. That's way too high maintenance for most of us. For more moderate at-home self-tanning, exfoliate in the shower every four or five days with a body scrub. Then just use a gradual tanning moisturizer every day or every other day.

4 **An expensive tan is just the base of beautiful skin.** The day of an important event, celebs finish off their skin with an illuminating product to complete the look. "The aim is healthy, glowing, luminous skin, not an artificial dark flat color," explains celebrity tanner Sophie Evans of St. Tropez Tan. These products, usually creams or lotions, are applied like makeup to areas like the collarbone, cleavage, shinbone, and down your biceps and calves to reflect light and attract attention. You can also use an illuminator to highlight a face tan, applying it on the tops of your cheekbones or mixing a little into your foundation to give your face a tan glow.

The Custom-Blended Tan

Here's how to get the tan Sophie Evans has given royalty, politicians, pop stars, and movie stars, a customized tan that looks better than the real thing.

1. YOU'LL NEED TWO TANNERS TO GET THE CUSTOM-BLENDED TAN LOOK:

A regular tanner that works for your skin tone: It's better to go lighter than darker, and keep in mind that choosing a tanner can be a little like choosing a man—you may have to kiss a few frogs before you find your prince.

A lighter tanner: Either a gradual self-tanner for the body, a facial self-tanner, or a diluted-down mixture of your regular tanner (half tanner to half oil-free moisturizer).

2. EXFOLIATE BEFORE YOU TAN, and every few days before reapplying, to remove dead cells and help fade the existing tan before you put on a new one.

3. TO PREVENT STREAKS, apply too much, not too little. Self-tanner is like paint, if you try to stretch a little amount over a large area, it will break and you'll see the wall. Apply liberally—any excess you can pat off with a soft towel or buffing mitt.

4. BEGIN WITH THE LARGE AREAS and lightly apply what's leftover to the smaller areas. Avoid applying too much self-tanner directly to the elbows, lower knees, wrists, fingers, and sides of feet. We'll get to those.

5. IF YOU SPRAY TAN YOURSELF AT HOME, Sophie recommends putting a towel on the floor and covering your feet with it: "When you spray, it all eventually goes down to your feet and they come out ten times darker," she says. At the end, take off the towel and give them one light spritz.

6. FOLLOW THE TIPS ON THE NEXT PAGE to tan your tricky parts so your tan doesn't look fake.

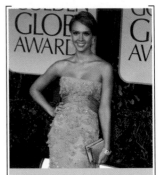

Jessica Alba's golden glow is crave-worthy.

Tanning Your Tricky Parts

These are the parts of your body that can make or break a self-tan. If you follow these directions you'll look flawless, not fake.

Hands
Because hands tend to get too dark and fade faster, the trick to a natural look is to use the diluted or lighter formula on them and blend well at the wrists and in between fingers. Always wipe the nails, cuticles, and palms with a cleansing wipe immediately after tanning to avoid any staining. Use the gradual tanner when hands start to fade, which will happen faster than on the rest of your body due to frequent washing.

Feet
Lots of women stop at the feet, leaving a line that looks like they're wearing footless hose. Using the diluted tanner or gradual tanner on the ankles and feet, blending it up to the ankle, is the trick here, too. Wipe toenails immediately to avoid any yellow staining, even if you're wearing nail polish. Last, always blend a little bit of moisturizer into creases that form when you move your feet to prevent tanner from catching in them.

Elbows, Ankles, Wrists, and Knees
Use the lighter formula or diluted formula on these areas, blending well where they meet your arms and legs. Or use your regular tanner and go over them about five minutes afterward with a thin coat of moisturizer to blend out any excess. Also blend moisturizer up the back of the heel and up the crease in the wrist to make the transitions seamless.

Inner Arms and Thighs
When arms and legs have a 360-degree tan it looks fake, so use a gradual tanner or diluted regular tanner (half tanner and half moisturizer) on inner arms and inner thighs where you wouldn't naturally get as much sun exposure.

Back
To do your back yourself, use an applicator mitt turned around the other way or apply product to the front of a gloved hand. Use a lot of product to make sure you cover everything, then use a soft towel to pat it down to remove excess. Sprays are also great for backs.

Face
A great face tan is almost like plastic surgery or long-lasting makeup—it can slim your chin, lift your cheekbones, and shade your eye sockets so your eye color pops, as well as conceal pimples and broken capillaries, and take the red out of skin. And because it lasts for a few days, it's a great thing to do before a long weekend when you don't want to have to wear makeup. The face has a tendency to go darker due to higher bacteria levels, so use a gradual facial tanner; diluting a tanner with moisturizer will help it from depositing into and darkening large pores.

BOOK AN APPOINTMENT WITH...

NICHOLA JOSS
The Celebrity Skin Finisher

You might think of gorgeous Nichola as a makeup artist for the body. She's at the forefront of the new skin-finishing trend, regularly both tanning and then "finishing" celeb skin the day of an event to produce the glowy, luminous, healthy look you admire on stars like Kate Moss, Scarlett Johansson, and Charlize Theron. Though ideally she'll tan a celeb a few days before and get to just enhance it at a shoot or for an event, she's also mastered a technique for body-baring emergencies you can use at home, which she shares on the opposite page.

TIPS FOR A GREAT-LOOKING TAN FOR A SPECIAL OCCASION

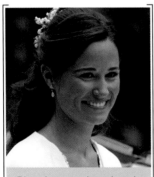

Pippa's tan at her sister's wedding took planning.

Back to Pippa and her sister, Kate, and their glowing golden bodies—these are the rules to follow to get a tan that looks royally hot, not heinous, for your own red-carpet or public appearance.

Tan two days before the event: Self-tanner can change on the skin after the first few days; having the tan applied two days prior gives it time to settle and adapt to your skin.

Do a test tan. You may need to go slightly deeper or slightly lighter depending on what you're wearing. Give yourself enough time to try on the dress two days later, like you would on the real occasion, to assess the true color.

If you want a darker tan, do what's referred to as a "double dip": a tan applied as single coats on two consecutive days.

THREE STEPS TO GORGEOUS GOING-OUT SKIN

by Nichola Joss

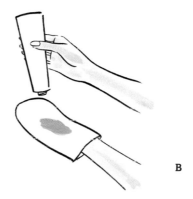

1. SKIN PREP. First use a dry body mitt to exfoliate, massaging it into all exposed body parts in circular motions, then applying moisturizer. (Sketch A)

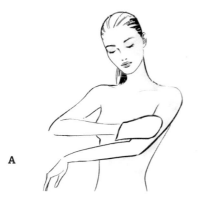

A

B

2. TUBE TAN. With the mitt, use a temporary tanner like St. Tropez's aptly named One Night Only. Joss is so confident this product won't transfer onto clothes, she's applied it right before the models walk the runway at shows for British designers Issa and Stella McCartney. (Sketch B)

3. ILLUMINATOR. Apply an illuminating cream, either gold-, silver-, pink-, or blue-based, to match your outfit or coloring, smoothing it on the front of the legs, down the center of arms, on collarbones, completely around the shoulder, and above the cleavage. (Sketch C)

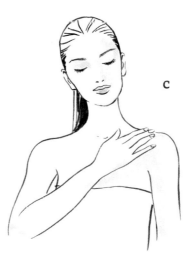

C

Andrea's Self-Tanning Tool Kit

MY FAVORITE TANNERS

—————— MOUSSE/LOTION ——————

SAVE

L'Oréal Paris Sublime Bronze Tinted Self-Tanning Lotion, $9.99
Fake Bake the Face Self-Tan Lotion, $23.95
Bare Escentuals Faux Tan Sunless Tanner, $22

SPLURGE

Clarins Delicious Self-Tanning Cream, $42
Lancôme Flash Bronzer Oil-Free Tinted Self-Tanning
Face Lotion with Vitamin E, $32
St. Tropez Self Tan Bronzing Mousse, $40

—————— TOWELETTE ——————

SAVE

L'Oréal Paris Sublime Bronze Self-Tanning Towelettes, $10.99

SPLURGE

Kate Somerville Somerville 360° Tanning Towelettes, $48

—————— GRADUAL ——————

SAVE

Jergens Natural Glow Revitalizing Daily Moisturizer, $8.49
Olay Quench Plus Touch of Sun Body Lotion, $8.99

SPLURGE

St. Tropez Gradual Tan Everyday Body, $30

——— SPRAY ———

SAVE

Neutrogena MicroMist Airbrush
Sunless Tan, $10.99

SPLURGE

Bliss A Tan for All Seasons, $36
St. Tropez Self Tan Bronzing Spray, $35

——— BODY ILLUMINATORS ———

SAVE

Physicians Formula Bronze Booster
Glow-Boosting Sun Stones, $14.95

SPLURGE

St. Tropez Bronzing Rocks, $40
St. Tropez Skin Illuminator, $22.50
Scott Barnes' Body Bling, $42

——— JUST-FOR-THE-NIGHT ———

SAVE

Sally Hansen Spray On Subtle Shimmer, $12.35

A liquid bronzer you already own
mixed with moisturizer, or moisturized legs
brushed with a powder bronzer

Fake Bake Bronze on the Glow, $17.95

SPLURGE

M·A·C Skinsheen Leg Spray, $26
(you can use it on any body skin)
St.Tropez Wash Off Instant Glow Mousse, $22.50

——— BODY MITTS ———

These cost less than $10 and are the real secret to
making a tan look rich—use them dry to exfoliate skin
before a tan or as an application tool for a streak-free
effect. "Using a mitt is what can give a tan that edgeless
finish," says Jennifer Aniston's tanner, Lucy Halperin.

St. Tropez Applicator Mitt, $6
Ulta Sunless Mitt, $4.99

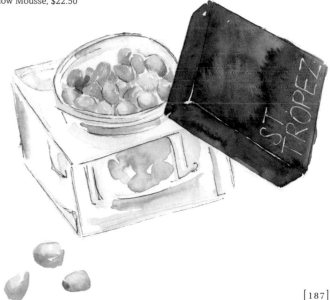

WHAT TO DO IF YOUR
TAN LOOKS CHEAP

Whether the color is off, it came out streaky, or you made an application mistake, you don't have to live with it. Here are a few ways to take off a tacky tan.

- **Mix lemon juice with baking soda into a paste,** then apply to the skin. Let sit five minutes, then take off with an exfoliating scrub or wipe. You'll need to experiment on your skin with a patch test to gauge the time to leave it on—no more than two or three minutes.

- **If it's a recently applied tan,** St. Tropez Tan Remover, $18, is genius. Works for the first four hours after applying.

- **Start over by doing a tan detox,** like St. Tropez Tan Detox, $35, to clear your skin of all color.

Phew! Looking well-kempt takes a lot of work!

If you can't afford to be high maintenance but want a high-maintenance grooming look, the best way to go is clean, natural, and well-cared for. Everything else is like tanning—icing on the cake. Pretty and natural always trumps artificial and fake. The key is to look like you take care of yourself without looking like that's all you care about. Got it? Let's review.

You Don't Have a Dime

- Brows that look like they are in a permanent state of surprise or shock

- Brows that look blocky and obviously made-up

- Rogue brow hairs that go unplucked

- Teeth so artificially white they could blind you . . . or just the opposite, teeth so stained, dull, or chipped it looks like you don't care about them

- A manicure that is on too long and/or nails with chipped polish or raggedy edges

- Dry, flaking cuticles and rough, scaly hands and feet

- Oops-I-forgot-to-shave legs or bikini line

- Ingrown hairs and bumps around your bikini line

- A tan that's too dark, too fake, or too obvious . . . you look like you fell in orange paint.

A Million Bucks

- Soft, perfectly arched brows that frame your face and accentuate your eyes

- Radiant, pearly white teeth that flash your excellent health and vitality along with your smile

- Nails with that just-left-the-salon look with high shine, a beautiful shape, and rich color, or at least nails that look clean, filed, shiny, and healthy if not polished

- Soft, touchable, hydrated skin

- Legs so smooth you can barely see a hair follicle, let alone stubble

- A bump-free (and hair-free) bikini line

- A glowing golden self-tan that looks better than the real thing

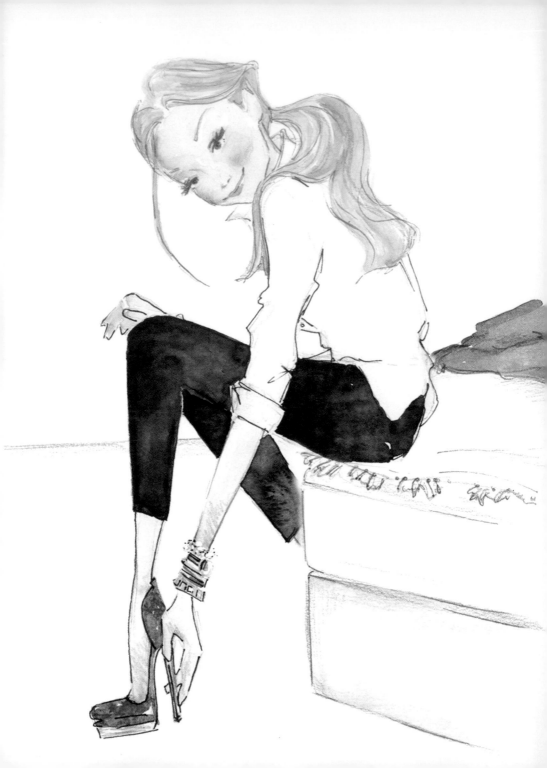

Pulling It All Together!

Fragance, Fashion, and a Review

By now you're on your way to getting the look you want—chic, modern, expensive—at a price you can afford. You know that looking expensive is about looking fresh and modern, not over-the-top or overdone, and that upgrading your look is more about having the knowledge, tips, tools, taste, and understanding to go for it than a wallet full of cash. But before we wrap things up and I send you on your way, there are a few more things we need to talk about that say eek instead of chic.

This chapter begins with fragrance, because wearing one that smells cheap—or wearing too much of even a beautiful one—is an instant turnoff. You won't have to bother with the rest of the book because no one will look at you anyway! Besides that, fragrance is a significant purchase, one you want to make smartly and wear appropriately. I'll show you how. Next, I touch on fashion with ten rules to live by that'll help you develop a chic, classic, individualized style. A hint: Stick with simple updates to classic shapes and basic colors, and wear your size, and you're halfway there. Finally, I'll pull it all together for you with a wrap-up of some of the important themes I want you to remember and turn to whenever you pull out this book or try out the advice inside. Frankly, I hope you'll think about them each time you buy a beauty product or get ready in front of the mirror for work or a party.

Fragrance

Another place where it's easy to cheapen your image and where less is always more. I think the scents that smell most expensive are those that smell fresh and natural, not too heavy, too sweet, or too powdery. A fragrance shouldn't enter the room before you do and it shouldn't make the whole room smell. It's meant to be something personal that only those who come really, really close to you notice. Even the world's most expensive perfume can smell as cheap and cloying as a car air freshener if you wear too much of it.

I think the scents that smell most expensive are those that smell fresh and natural, not too heavy, too sweet, or too powdery.

Make a Smart Fragrance Investment

Here's some advice from my go-to fragrance guru, Jessica Hanson, director of fragrances for Sephora:

- **It's not enough to like just the bottle and message of the fragrance.** "When you get to the heart of it, it's how it smells and how that impacts your brain that matters," she says.

- **Try a fragrance you're attracted to with your eyes closed.** Make sure you like the scent as much as you like the branding and bottle.

- **Always ask for samples.** Give your scent a trial run to be sure it doesn't offend anyone you love or work with before you buy it.

- **Start with a rollerball format of a fragrance.** These mini roll-on tubes cost less than $25 and are a great way to try out a pricey designer scent before making a bigger expenditure. Sephora offers sixty rollerballs that run the gamut from new releases to classy classics.

Remember, besides being the most expensive, perfume is the most intense form of fragrance. I don't even own any. Instead I usually wear the less pricey fragranced oils and lotion versions of my favorite scents for a more subtle effect that also subs as a body moisturizer. They're usually less expensive, the format dilutes the headiness, and the oil base makes them last longer on your body. Especially investment worthy are scented body lotions that contain treatment ingredients like antioxidants. If your favorite scent doesn't come in a lotion formula, you can mix a drop of perfume or one spritz of eau de toilette into a generous dollop of Jergens or Lubriderm in your hand and spread it all over your body.

> *I usually wear the less pricey fragranced oils and lotion versions of my favorite scents.*

Expensive Scent Application Tips

How you apply fragrance matters, too. It's so easy to
go overboard!

- **When I do apply eau de toilette,** I like to spray a little (and
  I mean a little, not a lot!) into the air in front of me and walk
  through it instead of spritzing it on pulse points—it makes
  for a more subtle effect.

- **Beauty heiress Aerin Lauder taught me this fragrance trick
  she learned from her grandmother Estée:** Spray the scent
  on your hairbrush. It'll cling to natural oils in your hair and
  make you smell delicious without overpowering.

- **If you do apply too much, use a baby wipe to take it off.**
  Don't add more—there's probably still enough lingering on
  your skin, even if you can no longer smell it.

- **Be careful about mixing too many scents at once.** Your
  hair products have a scent, your moisturizer probably has a
  scent, both of which may stand alone and make the need for
  a separate fragrance unnecessary. I can't tell you how many
  times I've gotten complimented on my fragrance when it
  was just my shampoo or the body oil I use on my legs.

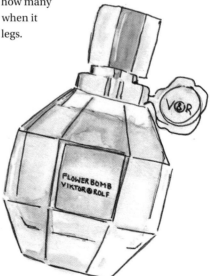

Couturize Your Fragrance

── PARK AVENUE PRETTY ──

Think modern luxe, sophisticated, pretty feminine florals with a hint of something unexpected, like a green, woody, or citrus note, to keep it sexy, not stuffy.
Try: *Dior Miss Dior or J'Adore, Chanel Chance Eau Tendre, Michael Kors, Pucci Miss Pucci*

── HOLLYWOOD BOHO ──

Go for natural-smelling green, citrusy, and fresh florals with unique notes.
Try: *Clean, Flower by Kenzo, Estée Lauder Sensuous Nude, Donna Karan Be Delicious, Philosophy Amazing Grace*

── GLAM GLOBE-TROTTER ──

Use a scent that takes you places with notes from exotic locales or vacation spots, fragrances that are casual but worldly.
Try: *Tocca fragrances, Tom Ford Violet Blonde, Thierry Mugler Alien*

── MODERN MOVIE STAR ──

Wear a bold, strong fragrance that's meant to get you noticed, with notes like orchid, jasmine, patchouli, and rose.
Try: *Viktor & Rolf Flowerbomb, Gucci Flora by Gucci, Tom Ford Black Orchid*

Fashion

Upgrading your beauty routine can overcome plenty but it won't compensate for certain wardrobe faux pas. Before I get into fashion that makes you look expensive and fashion that makes you look like you don't have a dime, I want to point out that I'm a real woman with the same fashion conundrums as you, who has to make the same kind of daily choices about what to wear when and what looks good on her body type.

Growing up in the fashion business (my family owned a famous dress company) with pretty stylish role models—my mom and stepmom have different styles but both always look impeccable and expensive, and having spent years working in magazines, I've watched and learned and tried out plenty of looks. What I've noticed is that looking expensive in your clothes doesn't mean you have to spend a fortune on them.

The kind of women who always look expensive are those who can make a dress from H&M look like a million bucks. I'm sure you know women who have the Midas touch with clothes. They look great no matter what they wear because they stick to a certain fashion formula that defies trends and always looks expensive, whether it comes from Prada or Target.

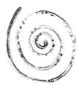

Andrea's Luxe Wardrobe Rules

1 **I stick to a basic color palette.** Whites, beiges, browns, navy, grays, and black—and jazz up my look by mixing in occasional jewel-tone-colored or print pieces in a shirt or jacket or a piece of jewelry.

2 **I collect statement jewelry, not diamonds.** Pieces with an exotic flair, like my favorite Thai gold necklace, or my geode or stone necklaces on beaded chains, these weren't very expensive but they make anything I wear look interesting and chic. Look for pieces like these on the street, at flea markets, in ethnic neighborhood stores, or when you travel. My jewelry designer friend Kara Ross makes a bridge collection of statement jewelry sold at department stores that'll give you this look for a lot less than her high-end collection (worn by stars and Michelle Obama). Talbots and J.Crew are also great places to find affordable statement jewelry, as is HSN.

3 **I spend money on accessories, not clothes.** A great pair of shoes or boots, belt, or scarf can add richness to even a T-shirt and jeans and last a lot longer. It's the opposite of the beauty spending I suggested, where I told you to spend money on the canvas (your skin care products, foundations) and save on the accessories (lipsticks, eye makeup).

4 **I pay attention to my undergarments.** I go for bra fittings once a year and buy a few new bras that really flatter my body and make my clothes look better. Most women think of themselves as having a certain bra size, but the reality is that your bra size changes from both hormones and weight gain or loss. And an ill-fitting or stretched-out bra can make your entire outfit look cheap. I've also got a nice collection of Spanx-like garments. They're not so sexy, but neither are bumps and bulges, and these are miracle workers. Most celebrities wear them—the trick is to be sure they don't play peekaboo, even when you sit down.

5 **When I do buy high-end designer, which is not that often, I don't wear it head to toe.** I especially avoid trendy pieces and patterns that will be recognizable as coming from a particular season. You don't want to be known as say, the Prada Girl or worse, the girl who wears last season's Prada. You want to be known as a girl who dresses beautifully and has a great fashion sense. Remember, labels that reek money, like highlights that are too obvious, make you look flashy (aka trashy!), like you're trying too hard or have no personal style (so you have to buy it).

6 **I'm best friends with my tailor.** This is something I learned from fashion designer Tory Burch. "The key to looking great is finding a tailor you trust and love. Everything looks better when it fits perfectly. Nipping a dress in at the waist or hemming a trouser so that it falls beautifully doesn't cost a lot, but it will transform your wardrobe," says Tory. Really, fit is everything—even if the tailor at the dry cleaner is the closest you'll get to haute couture.

7 **I like my shirts to have a three-quarters sleeve length.** It's flattering to most body shapes and lends a chic Audrey Hepburn look to clothes—slightly retro but totally modern.

8 **I'm a big fan of white shirts.** It doesn't matter if they're crisp white button-downs or long-sleeve white T-shirts. They look good in every season, year to year, and are versatile enough to wear to work, a party, over a bathing suit, or with jeans or a pair of slacks. And those statement necklaces look great with them!

Really, fit is everything—even if the tailor at the dry cleaner is the closest you'll get to haute couture.

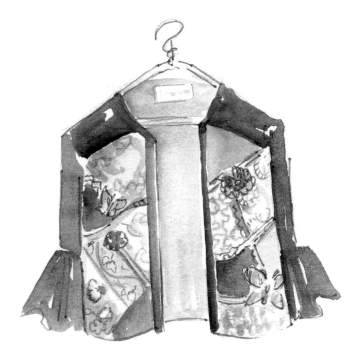

9 **I buy interesting one-of-a-kind jackets, dresses, and tops.** And then I incorporate them with basics to make a rich statement. For instance, I have one fun J. Mendel patchwork jacket with ruffle sleeves (sounds weird but it's gorgeous) that I bought at a sample sale that makes black pants and a black shirt from the Gap look like a designer outfit, and turns even the simplest black polyester dress into cocktail party material.

10 **I buy my size.** It's always more flattering to wear clothes that fit. And squeezing into ones that don't can make you look instantly tacky. Similarly, hiding your body in shapeless clothes doesn't do much for you, either. If a shirt, sweater, or dress seems too voluminous, I'll wear a simple skinny belt to add some shapeliness, something I learned from famed fashion stylist Mary Alice Stephenson.

The Wrap-Up!

Before I send you on your way, let's review some important themes you've heard over and over again throughout this book.

Less is always more. Cheap is often too much of a good thing. Simple looks classic; flashy looks trashy.

Build an edited beauty collection. By choosing the right products, you'll need less . . . and spend less.

Knowledge is priceless. If you know what you want and how to get it, you can DIY. If you're an informed client, you'll get your money's worth at the salon, makeup counter, dermatologist, or nail spa.

Price point isn't as important as good taste. All the money in the world can't buy taste, but once you develop good taste, you can find it for any price.

Maintenance is everything. Remember that a cheap manicure is a good manicure that's been on too long.

Expensive-looking hair and makeup doesn't advertise itself. It's understated, refined, tasteful, not blingy. It makes you look like the best version of yourself, not like somebody else.

Buying new beauty products is a lot cheaper than buying new clothes—and you'll get more wear out of them. A new lipstick, eyeliner, or especially nail polish is a way to accessorize your existing wardrobe and feel fresh and stylish without stepping into a fitting room.

The key to a look that reads high net worth is to enhance what you've got without trying to be someone else. "You, only better" is the goal of each and every tip and technique you've read about in this book.

THE FREEBIES!

There are a few things that can make you look instantly more expensive that don't cost a dime—and they're all interrelated.

Good posture: Standing up straighter makes you look taller, thinner, and more confident.

A smile: When you smile, you radiate confidence and self-worth.

Self-confidence: It's all about believing in yourself. If you don't feel it, fake it . . . stand up straighter and smile!

I hope I've educated you on the looks you want, the ones that make you look like a million bucks, and the mistakes that can bankrupt your look. And now that you know the difference between the two, you'll use this book as a guide to help you get it right when you DIY in your bathroom mirror or head out to purchase a beauty product or service. Take your time and try these tips one at a time. This book is meant to be a resource to help you make major changes that will upgrade your look to upgrade your life.

I promise, if you put in the time and make smart beauty choices like the ones I've shared with you, you'll reap the benefits. Because as I've preached to you throughout this book, when you look good, you feel good. And when you feel good, you'll radiate an aura of beauty confidence that will attract attention and help you get what you want out of life, be it a promotion, a better job, a loving relationship, or whatever it is that makes you feel content and complete. Truly. Investing in yourself, unlike an investment in the stock market, is a guaranteed win-win, bound to pay off, as long as you go in as an informed consumer and make the right choices. Now it's up to you to go for it!

When you feel good, you'll radiate an aura of beauty confidence.

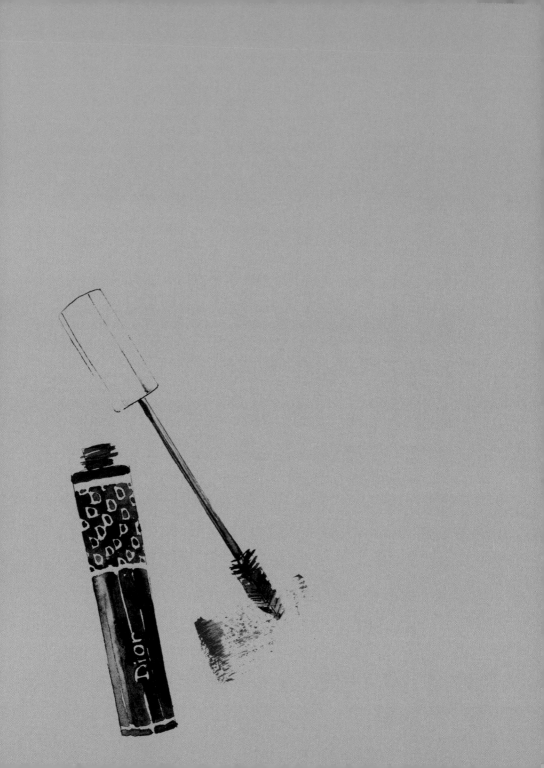

BEAUTY REFERENCES AND RESOURCES

These are some of my favorite resources for finding beauty inspiration, buying and researching products, getting good prices and extra benefits, and booking beauty services at the best price possible.

Online Beauty Shopping

Drugstore.com & Beauty.com
Great sites for all kinds of beauty products, mass and prestige; if you register as a member you'll get constant discount offers.

Amazon.com/beauty
I like Amazon for researching products and reading reviews.

Sephora.com
Become a beauty insider to get loads of special offers.

Ulta.com
A great mix of high-end, mass-market, and salon brands in the same place; register for great discounts.

Folica.com
This site is run by self-proclaimed "hair junkies" and has great deals on everything from styling tools to specialty shampoos.

Dermstore.com
Founded by a board-certified dermatologist, this site is chock-full of reviews and you get free shipping and free samples with every order.

SallyBeauty.com
One of the world's largest beauty-supply retailers, this is a great place to get salon-quality tools for home use at excellent prices.

RickysNYC.com
An eclectic New York beauty-supply store where you can find the latest trends, like argon-oil infused combs, as well as cult classics and hard-to-find professional items, like the bungee cords for making ponytails. I love all their brushes.

BeautyBar.com
BeautyBar.com offers the same free two-day shipping as Soap.com, but specializes in the world's top luxury brands, including both well-known and up-and-coming collections. What people love most about this site is the customer service; if you don't like something you can send it back and the BeautyBar team is available 24-7 to answer any questions.

LovelySkin.com
This site sells thousands of skin care products you can often find only at dermatologists' and plastic surgeons' offices, and it's owned and run by Dr. Joel Schlessinger, a top dermatologist who often personally recommends products and responds to customer questions.

QVC.com/beauty
A great option for buying kits and single items from brands like Laura Geller, Mally, Bobbi Brown, Tarte, and more. You'd be surprised at the high-end brands that offer specially priced kits and deals on QVC!

Beauty.HSN.com
Look for savings on cult brands like Deborah Lippmann (New York Fashion Week's polish queen) and Carol's Daughter, a natural line designed to work on a diverse range of skin types and tones.

RMSBeauty.com
Organic makeup from Rose-Marie Swift, a top makeup artist with clients like Eva Mendes, Gisele, and Miranda Kerr. I love her Living Luminizer highlighter. A must-have!

Birchbox.com
Get four to five deluxe beauty samples from some of the top brands in the industry for $10/month. It's like the birthday gift that never stops.

DollarNailArt.com
The largest selection of nail art supplies on the Internet, and the best part is, everything is a dollar, including great foil nail overlays that are easy to apply yourself and a favorite of top celebrity manicurists.

VapourBeauty.com
Award-winning organic makeup created by a young breast cancer survivor.

CND.com
Head to Creative Nail Design's main website to find a certified Shellac salon near you. Be sure to check out the Fashion Week and the Style Look Book each season for a recap of the hottest nail trends.

GoIndulge.com
Great resource for buying CND nail care products online.

Bumbleandbumble.com
On this genius site, you can browse different hair looks by length and peruse the Bb.Buzz section for an inside look at their hairstyles from Fashion Week.

TotalBeauty.com
Trustworthy beauty reviews on a variety of products, ranging from drugstore to prestige, to help you research before you buy.

Beauty Services Deal Sites

Lifebooker.com
New York City–based beauty deal site that offers up to 70 percent off top beauty treatments like gel manicures, Botox, and even massages.

Groupon.com
Even though you might not think to check out the beauty deals on this popular online discount destination, the quality of local services at great prices will surprise you!

LivingSocial.com
Check out the "Families" and "Nationwide Deals" tabs for beauty bargains.

GiltCity.com
The vouchers offered on this site get you into some of the top spas and salons in the country.

StyleSeat.com
This site lets you shop for a stylist at home. You can view individual websites from thousands of stylists in your area and book an appointment.

Reference and Inspiration

MakeupAlley.com
Also known as MUA, this huge database of member-generated product reviews and message boards is where you can discover underground beauty goods and priceless tips.

Pinterest.com
Check out the hair and beauty boards for pictorial step-by-step looks for hair, makeup, and nails, as well as links to beauty blog posts and videos and inspirational photos of looks to try.

AllLacqueredUp.com
A nail-trend blog jam-packed with nail tips, tricks, and advice.

GreenYourBeauty.com
Wonderful tips to "green" your beauty routine and reviews on natural cosmetic products.

Temptalia.com
This beauty blog has fan favorite features like the Makeup Dupe List, Swatch Gallery, and the Makeup Recommendations List that help you find less-expensive look-alikes of high-end products.

Intothegloss.com
Features insider advice from fashion and beauty influencers.

M•A•C makeup artist Twitter feeds
The brand's pro artists tweet about their work during Fashion Week. It's fascinating and full of tips.

NARS Twitter feed (@NARSissist)
Includes info on new product launches and offers precious tips for using NARS products.

Glamour.com newsletter
I started it and it remains a great way to have excellent, usable beauty tips delivered right to your inbox.

EsteeLauder.com/GuestBlogger
Cleverly written by Emily Schuman of the blog *Cupcakes and Cashmere*, this is a great

resource for trend breakdowns and tutorial videos.

BeautyBloggingJunkie.com
This hilarious blog is headed by Amber Katz and includes interviews, Q&As with top makeup artists, and product reviews.

ShakeYourBeauty.com
Tia Williams, the former beauty editor at Essence.com and successful author, keeps her posts interesting with heartwarming and hilarious anecdotes.

Afrobella.com
Self-described as a "continual celebration of natural hair and women of all shades of beautiful," Patrice Grell Yursik offers priceless advice on all things beauty.

BeautyBlitz.com
This online beauty magazine was started by former editors from *InStyle* and *Marie Claire* and has regular features like "Celebrity Editors" with posts from chic celebs like Chanel Iman and Bar Refaeli, and "Beauty Stalkers," which profiles movers and shakers in the beauty business.

DailyMakeover.com
Keep up to date on celeb makeovers with plenty of before and after photos on this site, then head to the Virtual Makeover to begin your own transformation.

CelebrityHairColorGuide.com
A site that reveals hair color formulas to create looks like top celebrities. Share this site with your colorist!

EWG.org
The Environmental Working Group's Skin Deep Cosmetics Database lets you check the ingredients of almost every cosmetic and personal-care product on the market and provides you with safety ratings.

Tutorials

St. Tropez Tanning Tips, www.StTropezTan.com/application-videos
Tips and how-to videos from the United Kingdom's top tanning company that celebs swear by.

BeautyVT.com/Category/Hair
Professional how-tos from former Aveda creative director

Jon Reyman. It's meant to teach real women what the pros know. It's like having a stylist in your own bathroom!

YouTube.com
Great makeup tips from Michelle Phan, pixiwoo, Panacea81 (Lauren Luke), and Kandee Johnson.

MakeupGeek.com
A collection of celebrity-inspired, beginner-focused advanced hair and makeup video lessons.

TheBeautyDepartment.com
Chic, simple, and hip beauty tutorials with inspirational photos, lifestyle advice, and beauty tips mixed in.

Aveda.com video library
Fabulous hair care and makeup how-to videos.

Fekkai.com
Head to "Backstage with Fekkai" for runway inspiration and Fashion Week videos.

BobbiBrown.com/Learn
Articles, videos, and tips from Bobbi and her team.

Shopping for Chic Clothing and Accessories

V by Eva on HSN
Inexpensive clothing and accessories designed by Eva Jeanbart-Lorenzotti, founder of the upscale and very chic e-commerce website Vivre.com.

Kara Ross NY
Less expensive line from Kara Ross, a contemporary jewelry designer whose signature collection is a celebrity and editorial favorite. Still not cheap, but amazing pieces that'll make anything you wear them with, even a plain T-shirt, instantly chic.

Carol Brodie's Rarities Collection on HSN
Fine jewelry at great prices from a former Harry Winston celebrity jewelry expert.

Shopafrolic.com
Great fashion inspiration and low-cost alternatives to high-end looks from my good friends, the genius sisters Liz Lange and Jane Steinberg.

Shoplatitude.com
Unique style finds from all over the world. I love this site for exotic jewelry and handbags, the kind I seek out when I travel—without a plane ticket!

Net-A-Porter.com
Check out their unbelievable sales on high-end fashion items and become a member so you don't miss the sale notifications. Check out TheOutnet.com, Net-A-Porter's sister discount site; think of it as a luxury clothing outlet, but without the lines!

Rue La La
Members are offered exclusive access to private sale boutiques in the fashion, home, and beauty categories.

ToryBurch.com
Head to "The Tory Blog" for style tips, best-dressed lists, and even advice on where to shop and eat around the country.

My "Book an Appointment with" Experts

I can't thank all my beauty BFFs enough for their incredible contributions to this book. All were willing to share their best tips, exclusive secrets, and techniques with me, providing hundreds of thousands of dollars of beauty advice to all of you, and I can't thank them enough for it.

Adir Abergel
www.starworksartists.com
/news/category/tag/
adir abergel

David Babaii
www.traceymattingly.com
/hair/david-babaii

Creighton Bowman
CreightonBowman.com

Harry Josh
HarryJosh.com

Oscar Blandi
OscarBlandi.com

Sharon Dorram
SharonDorram.com

Doug Macintosh
www.facebook.com/pages
/Doug-MacintoshCelebrity
-Hair-Colorist/69252065196

Tracey Cunningham
www.facebook.com
/pages/Tracey-Cunningham
/59857941094

Dr. David Colbert
ColbertMD.com

Nerida Joy
NeridaJoySkincare.com and
BeautyMint.com

Dr. Bobby Buka
BobbyBukaMD.com

Stacy Cox
www.StacyCoxTVHost.com
/index.asp

Talia Shobrook
www.taliashobrook.tumblr
.com

Romy Soleimani
www.ManagementArtists
.com/hair-makeup/
romy-soleimani

Laura Geller
LauraGeller.com

Jeffrey Paul
www.facebook.com
/pages/Jeffrey-Paul
-Beauty/125147237537373

Kimmie Kyees
KimmieKNails.com

Lidia Tivichi
www.Marisdusan.com

Nichola Joss
www.StTropezTan.com
/expertadvice

More Beauty BFFs

These experts contributed amazing tips, techniques, and their expensive advice throughout this book.

Gita Bass, Nick Barose, Kim Bower, Bobbi Brown, Tory Burch, Kelsey Deenihan, Giada De Laurentiis, Sophie Evans, Frédéric Fekkai, Brett Freedmam, Katherine Goldman, Lucy Halperin, Jessica Hanson, Ole Henriksen, Chanel Iman, Aerin Lauder, Jeanine Lobell, Dr. Ellen Marmur, Tracie Martyn, Julie Morgan, Dr. Sheldon Nadler, Olivia Palermo, George Papanikolas, Paul Podlucky, Kara Ross, Vanessa Scali, Dr. Irwin Smigel, Kate Somerville, Jin Soon Choi, Mary Alice Stephenson, Rose-Marie Swift, Luba Tadova, Amy Tagliamonti, Roxanne Valinoti, Bobby Wells, Dr. Jessica Wu

PHOTOGRAPHY CREDITS

4 Kate Middleton: David Jones/WPA Pool/Getty Images. 4 Gwyneth Paltrow: J.B Nicholas/Splash News/Newscom. 4 Natalie Portman: AP Images. 5 Zoe Saldana: Steve Granitz/WireImage/Getty Images. 5 Taylor Swift: Frazer Harrison/Getty Images. 5 Nicole Richie: JB Lacroix/WireImage/Getty Images. 6 Angelina Jolie: James Devaney/WireImage/Getty Images. 6 Kate Winslet: Dave Hogan/Getty Images. 6 Georgina Chapman: Jamie McCarthy/Getty Images. 7 Sandra Bullock: Lester Cohen/WireImage/Getty Images. 7 Penelope Cruz: JMAB/VMAB WENN Photos/Newscom. 7 Reese Witherspoon: Jeff Vespa/WireImage/Getty Images. 15 Angelina Jolie: MARCOCCHI GIULIO/SIPA/Newscom. 17 Anne Hathaway: Amanda Leddy/Splash News/Newscom. 19 Gwyneth Paltrow: Mike Marsland/WireImage/Getty Images. 21 Ellen Pompeo: AP Images. 23 Julianna Margulies: Casey Rogers/NBC Universal/Getty Images. 32 Jessica Alba: Todd Oren/WireImage/Getty Images.

34 Sienna Miller: Mike Marsland/WireImage/Getty Images. 38 Nicole Richie: Michael Tran/FilmMagic/Getty Images. 38 Sofia Vergara: Jordan Strauss/WireImage/Getty Images. 38 Blake Lively: Jason Merritt/Getty Images. 39 Kate Winslet: AP Images. 39 Kate Hudson: Fitzroy Barrett/ZUMAPRESS/Newscom. 38 Beyoncé Knowles: John Sciulli /WireImage/Getty Images. 42 Emma Watson: AP Images. 42 Olivia Palermo: Richie Buxo/Splash News/Newscom. 42 Kate Middleton: Matt Baron/Getty Images. 42 Michelle Williams: Jeff Frank/ZUMA Press/Newscom. 42 Emily Blunt: George Pimentel/WireImage/Getty Images. 42 Olivia Wilde: Jen Lowery/Splash News/Newscom. 43 Carey Mulligan: Neil Mockford/FilmMagic/Getty Images. 43 Heidi Klum: John Lamparski/Getty Images. 43 Angelina Jolie: Lester Cohen/WireImage/Getty Images. 43 Scarlett Johansson: Steve Granitz/WireImage/Getty Images. 43 Reese Witherspoon: Nate Beckett/Splash News/Newscom. 43 Rosie Huntington-Whiteley:

Jamie McCarthy/WireImage/Getty Images. 44 Zoe Saldana: Getty, Steve Granitz/WireImage/Getty Images. 44 Emma Stone: Jordan Strauss/WireImage/Getty Images. 44 Olivia Wilde: Christopher Polk/ VF12/Getty Images. 50 Blake Lively: INB WENN Photos/Newscom. 50 Julia Roberts: SIPA via AP Images. 53 Jessica Biel: Carlos Alvarez/Getty Images. 53 Ashley Greene: Matt Carr/Getty Images. 54 Julianne Moore: Vera Anderson/WireImage/Getty Images. 60 Minka Kelly: Gary Gershoff/WireImage/Getty Images. 62 Gwyneth Paltrow: AP Images. 62 Chanel Iman: DB5 WENN Photos/Newscom. 62 Jessica Chastain: Julien Hekimien/Getty Images. 62 Carey Mulligan: AP Images. 62 Rachel Bilson: Venturelli/WireImage/Getty Images. 62 Christina Hendricks: AO1 WENN Photos/Newscom. 63 Gisele Bündchen: S. Granitz/WireImage/Getty Images. 63 Freida Pinto: David Thompson/ FilmMagic/Getty Images. 63 Julianne Moore: Mike Coppola/Getty Images. 63 Diane Kruger: NIVIERE/SIPA/Newscom.

ACKNOWLEDGMENTS

I've always wanted to write a book, but it was **Debra Goldstein** who finally got me to do it. Your encouragement of my idea from the minute I shared it with you over one of our many breakfasts at Le Pain is what got this project going.

To **Jessica Sindler,** my stylish and devoted editor at Gotham with the great eye makeup and stunningly chic casual updos, I thank you for believing in the project from the very start, for your guidance, excellent editing skills, always available ear, and dedication and patience to make this book live up to my vision of it. To **Lauren Marino, Bill Shinker, Sabrina Bowers, Erica Ferguson, Lindsay Gordon, Casey Maloney, Monica Benalcazar,** and everyone at Gotham who helped bring *How to Look Expensive* to life and out into the world. I am so grateful.

A huge thank you and so much gratitude to the very talented **Eric Hoffman** at Hoffman Creative, who believed in me from the very first phone call. I am so grateful for the beautiful work you and your fabulous team of **Tracy Engelhardtsen** and **Tamara McCarthy-Mayoral** have done to bring my words and advice alive on these pages.

I was lucky enough to be introduced to the fabulous up-and-coming fashion illustrator **Dallas Shaw** by my friends at Beneville Studios. Dallas' beautiful illustrations grace the advertising of some of the world's top luxury brands, such as Chanel, Ralph Lauren, and DKNY, and I am so honored to have her gorgeous, whimsical illustrations of me in this book. To **Aimee Levy,** for expertly creating the how-to sketches in this book. Thank you. To **Laura Wyss** for all your efforts to find the perfect photos. And big thanks to the very talented fresh out of Penn intern **Kimberly Eisler** and **Al Filreis** of Kelly Writers House for sending her to me!

I don't even know how to thank **Molly Adams,** my trusted assistant and so much more. This project owes so much to your smarts, dedication, and ability to do it all, whether that meant coming up with the perfect caption, deciphering the directions for a haircut and researching the ideal photo to represent it, pulling me out of my most challenging moment of writer's block, or cooking the most delicious, healthy dinner. I am so thankful to have your talent, warmth, grace, and strength be a part of my book and my life. You really have been my partner on this book, and I can't wait to someday celebrate your first cookbook! I also can't thank **Shirley Cover** and **Marita Santiago** enough for all their help, always, from keeping things organized to trying on lipsticks and blush and so much more.

To **Larry Shire** and **Jonathan Ehrlich** at Grubman, Indursky & Shire. You both just got *How to Look Expensive* from the moment you read the proposal. I so appreciate your wisdom and advice.

To my friends at *Glamour*: **Cindi Leive** for writing the beautiful foreword of this book and always being an advocate of my work and ideas, **Lauren Brody,** Deputy Editor, for always embracing my ideas and helping me improve on them, **Felicia Milewicz** and **Mary MacLean,** both of whom I've worked with forever and have helped shaped my ideas about beauty from the very beginning.

To all my friends in the beauty world for all your support throughout my career. Though I can't mention you all, a special thanks to **Jacquie Tractenberg, Alison Brod, Harris Shepard, Suzie Fleischman, Jan Arnold, Julia Labaton, Evan Miller, Leslie Stevens, William Lauder, Jane Hertzmark, John Dempsey, Susan Hageman, Diane Falcone, Tina Thomson, Laura Geller,** and

Scott Yardley. Your support of this book and my career is so appreciated.

To **Alison Mazzola** and her team, thank you for your friendship, advice, and for welcoming me into your office space. **Vanessa Discrio, Suze Yalof, Mary Alice Stephenson, Tory Burch, Kara Ross,** you are all my style gurus.

A big thank you to my own beauty team. **Sharon Dorram,** who keeps my hair gold-card gorgeous; **Antoinette Beenders** and **Karmela Lozina** for their genius haircuts; **Nella Talaba** from Sharon Dorram's Upper East Side Townhouse for her excellent blow-dries and life advice; **Demetris** and the entire team at the chic little DS Studio, my go-to neighborhood salon; **Jin Soon Choi** and her staff for the world's best manicures; **Luba Tadova** at Laura Geller Studio for her great makeup, lash and brow work; **Julie Morgan,** makeup artist/friend/advice guru, who did my makeup for my author picture and many a special occasion; dermatologists **Ellen Marmur, David Colbert, Debra Jaliman,** for taking my personal calls as well as my professional ones.

And a huge thank you to all my beauty friends who contributed to this book (see Beauty References and Resources section for a full listing).

To my friends at TCPW at Penn and CPW here in New York. You're the sororities I never had and your friendships both professionally and personally add so much value to my life.

To all my friends, both in New York and Nantucket—where I buckled down and finished up this book—for your patience, support, understanding, and cheerleading of me and this book.

To the late beauty icons **Evelyn Lauder** and **Charla Krupp,** both of whom passed while I wrote this book, you both so inspired me and taught me so much throughout my career. I also want to acknowledge **Geri Fessler,** a cousin who also lost her cancer battle last year. Geri's motto—live, love, laugh—and her love of sparkly makeup (that never looked cheap) will not be forgotten. I know she was looking forward to reading this book and I hope her daughters will enjoy and learn from it. Finally, to **Helen Gurley Brown,** my unforgettable boss during the nineties, for teaching me to always "Go for it." There's no such thing as a free lunch. Hard work gets you everywhere. Helen, your wisdom inspires how I live my life every day.

As I said in the dedication of this book, the biggest beauty secret of all is surrounding yourself with love, and for that I have my family to thank: **Mimi** and **Sandy Furman, Laura** and **John Pomerantz, Barbara Lustig, Susie Davis, Marnie** and **Neil Maclean** and all the Lustigs, Davises, and Orels, I am forever grateful for your love and support while I wrote this book and each and every day.

Matthew, it's finally your turn. You are my life partner, my rock, my best friend, my everything. I especially love your support of this project even when it got in the way of our life. **Anna,** as I said in the dedication, this book is for you. It's filled with so much that I've learned throughout my career and I hope it will be your beauty bible. **Michael,** I know you've said I'm just a beauty editor (not qualified to edit a middle school paper!) but despite that, I know you're proud of what I've accomplished and I hope watching me go through this process will inspire you to put your heart into whatever it is you love. That's why I devote so much of my time to the three of you! **James,** you are so filled with love and passions. I hope you see that being a beauty writer and editor is one of my passions, not just an attempt to waste time on the computer! Thank you ALL!

ABOUT THE AUTHOR

Andrea Pomerantz Lustig is known around the offices of *Glamour* as the "Beauty Sleuth," thanks to the wildly popular beauty advice column and articles she's written for the magazine for the last decade, as well as her BlackBerry bursting with the hottest beauty pros. She started Glamour.com's beauty blog and is cherished by *Glamour* readers for her fresh, original beauty tips, ideas, and solutions. Prior to becoming a contributing editor at *Glamour,* she was pioneer editor in chief at Sephora.com, and before that she spent ten years as beauty and fitness director at *Cosmopolitan.* She regularly appears in the national media, on shows including *The Early Show, Good Morning America, Today, Oprah*, and *Entertainment Tonight.* Her beauty tips have appeared in *Glamour, The New York Times, Women's Wear Daily, Allure,* and bloggers share her tips with their audiences regularly. A graduate of the University of Pennsylvania, she lives in New York City with her husband and three children.

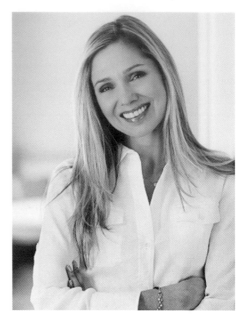